Emotional Care of Hospitalized Children

Emotional Care
of Hospitalized Children

An Environmental Approach

Madeline Petrillo, R.N., M.Ed.

Mental Health Consultant to Pediatric Nursing,
New York Hospital–Cornell Medical Center

and

Sirgay Sanger, M.D.

Clinical Assistant Professor in Child Psychiatry,
New York Hospital–Cornell Medical Center

J. B. LIPPINCOTT COMPANY

Philadelphia • Toronto

Copyright © 1972, By J. B. Lippincott Company

This book is fully protected by copyright and, with the exception of brief excerpts for review, no part of it may be reproduced in any form by print, photoprint, microfilm, or by any other means without the written permission of the publishers.

Distributed in Great Britain by
Blackwell Scientific Publications
Oxford ● London ● Edinburgh

ISBN Paperbound: 0—397—54124—4
ISBN Clothbound: 0—397—54126—0
Library of Congress Catalog Card Number 74—171534

Printed in the United States of America

Library of Congress Cataloging in Publication Data

Petrillo, Madeline, 1935-
    Emotional care of hospitalized children.

    1. Children—Hospital care. 2. Child mental
health. I. Sanger, Sirgay, 1935-   joint author.
II. Title.
RJ242.P47   610.73'62   74-171534

ISBN-0-397-54126-0
ISBN-0-397-54124-4 (pbk.)

To Our Parents

and to

Terry and Vicky

Preface

In our work with children, parents, and staff, we have evolved, through trial and error, a comprehensive program that applies theory to improving the lot of children who become hospitalized.

In seeing the effects of hospitalization on children, we thought there was a need for an explicit guide-in-depth of just how to deal with the common problems: (a) of the effects of severe stress, and (b) of every-day coping abilities of children and parents. This exposition is divided into major areas that coalesce into a health promoting milieu. These areas are: a general knowledge of growth and development, the forces of family and culture, human reactions to stress, loss and separation. Also, preventive approaches that have the effect of minimizing trauma to children and their families are given in the form of our actual protocols.

Rationale for this presentation is to bridge the gap between understanding and action. This book offers a practical, essential knowledge and its direct application without sacrificing the subtlety and sophistication that have been acquired over the past 30 years by many individual workers in these disciplines.

This book is intended for all those who have a part in the clinical management of children, and for those professionals who see in the instance of a child's hospitalization, an opportunity for promotion of growth, health and maturity. Specifically, it should prove to be beneficial to medical students, house officers, pediatricians, nurses, student nurses, psychiatric liaison, child psychiatry residents, hospital administrators, clinical psychology students, dietitians, recreation workers, hospital teachers, social workers and student social workers. Sections should be useful as manuals for the technique of communicating with children, other sections for the instruction of parents. Finally, the book supports a systems theory approach to helping children that is implied throughout by the emphasis on the interplay of dynamisms, individually and collectively. Clinical vignettes graphically illustrate the successes and failures of the work.

MADELINE PETRILLO, R.N., M.ED.
SIRGAY SANGER, M.D.

Acknowledgments

The authors are grateful for the support of Muriel Carbery whose imagination at the outset and continuous interest made possible the implementation of their ideas.

The following staff members' participation in the earliest months of the program ensured its later success: Alice DonDero, Carol Hanna, Judith Moore, Elda Bertagna, Giorgia Bryer, Judy Gennaro, Joan Callahan, Marie Monaco, Patricia Jennings, Judy Page, Judith Descoteau, Mary Watkins, Deanna Kelly, Doris Hyncik, Sharon Stubblefield, Sue Block, Mary Hogan, Sandra Morris, Christina Emru, Eleanor Fiori, Janet Powers, Patricia Prendergast, Claire Tangvold, Eleanor Landsman, Peter Auld, Barbara Ashe, Alan DeMayo, William Seed, Irving Kolin, Fred Kleinberg.

Special appreciation is given to the assistants in the mental health program: Page Kelly and Sally Everson.

Some of the liaison work described herein had its first trial in the Children's Unit of the Massachusetts Mental Health Center, The Children's Hospital in Boston, and the Child Psychiatry Department of the Massachusetts General Hospital—in the early 1960's. Inspirational teachers and instructors at these three hospitals were: Gregory Rochlin, Donald Gair, Elizabeth Zetzel, Elvin Semrad, Charles Pinderhughes, Christopher Standish, Aydin Ciankardas, Richard Peebles, John Lamont, Richard Galdston, Harold Stalvey, Margaret Bullowa, John Nemiah, Carl Binger, and Suzanne van Amerongen.

Contents

7. Loss, Grief and Death

8. The Mental Health Team in Action 213

Introduction

Although today we are quite sophisticated regarding the psychological responses of children to illness and hospitalization, it is striking to note the discrepancies between what we know and what we practice in the hospital environment. Indeed, we need to know more, and we need to encourage more research. But, at this time, it is our belief that the most compelling need is for the application of existing knowledge by those most intimately involved in patient care.

With few exceptions, the policies and routines of the majority of pediatric departments in this country are little different from those of the pediatric departments of several decades ago. Research findings have brought about drastic changes in physical treatment but have had only minimal influence on the total care of the patient. It is our overall philosophy that only by being prepared to utilize available knowledge in the many aspects of child development can we be of greatest service to children, who by the occasion of illness, present us with an extraordinary opportunity to look beyond the immediate sickness to their general adaptation.

Early study in child behavior was oriented toward sickness. Thus, conclusions were presented in the language of pathology, rather than in terms of adaptation. Characteristically, theories expressed in psychiatric jargon were clear to a select few, and so failed to reach a wide audience.

As the normal child became the subject of study, the situation appeared more hopeful. Paramedical personnel—nurses, social workers, physical and recreational therapists—were more frequently exposed to courses in the behavioral sciences. Still, this exposure was not reflected in child care practices. Theories were not yet translated into practical techniques applicable to hospitalized children. There has been little in the behavior of professionals to indicate their having had special education in human development.

Skilled personnel from various disciplines, working independently, have attempted to promote a comprehensive approach to child management,

1

but they have found it difficult to affect permanent change without the wide support of colleagues. Others, such as volunteers or students, have succeeded in working creatively with individual children, but were able to make only fleeting impressions on the field. For instance, the study by Prugh, et al., on the emotional reactions of children and families to hospitalization, which should be considered a classic, was published in the *American Journal of Orthopsychiatry* in January, 1953, and is now completely unfamiliar to medical and nursing personnel in the 1970's. Under these circumstances only a few have benefited from an altered approach to child care.

What has not occurred is a change in the basic philosophy of most pediatric departments to affect the total environment for hospitalized children. This change is accomplished only with administrative support.

A change in the environment requires that the permanent pediatric staff of all disciplines be educated in the application of theory; that they become sensitive to the meaning of hospitalization and treatment to children; that they develop communication skills and techniques for working constructively with children and their families and that they utilize their understanding of growth and development to identify problems that are present before hospitalization, as well as those induced by illness. Specifically, they need to know how to work with particular age groups, how to interpret medical/surgical conditions and treatment. They need to know ways to help children master the stresses of hospitalization and how to recognize obstacles to optimal health. Our thesis is that professionals in child care ought to know as much about the mind as the body.

With this background, pediatric personnel become the role models who are able to indicate to new personnel how to intervene in certain situations. They point to the kind of approach which is valued and rewarded. In short, they demonstrate the application of mental health concepts into skills that can be applied in tangible ways to child care. Until this occurs we will see a continuation of existing practices; that is, the arbitrary and disease-oriented management of patients.

How can the lag between our understanding and our actions be bridged if not by focusing directly upon the problem? This book is an attempt to do just this by describing one program designed to create a therapeutic environment for the care of hospitalized children.

Origins

To understand the current program, it is important to examine its beginnings. It evolved from two classic disciplines—nursing and psychiatry—and developed into an entity distinctly its own, while retaining basic characteristics of each and expanding to include other disciplines.

FROM THE PERSONAL POINT OF VIEW OF THE NURSING MENTAL HEALTH CONSULTANT

My interest in total child care began with my experience as an instructor in pediatric nursing. During this period, I was impressed with the ease of communicating to young students the essential needs of hospitalized children—both the physical and emotional. In the clinical area, students demonstrated eagerness and ability to apply classroom instruction. However, it was obvious that with their departure, clinical practice returned to the usual emphasis on physical treatment rather than on the care of the whole child.

I was disappointed to note that many of the same students returning to pediatrics as new graduates no longer functioned on the same level. In their initial encounters with sick children, they received the guidance and support of their instructors. At that time, teachers' values were most influential. Students also received grades for their ability to attain course objectives. In the roles of new staff members, however, they encountered a different set of values—all indisputably important. Priorities were efficiency in carrying out procedures, along with managerial and organizational skills.

Rewards for perpetuating the system and imitating established role models were made tangible by professional advancement and social acceptance. In this setting a child-centered approach to medical care failed to flourish; not because it was overtly discouraged, but simply because it was not highly regarded, and so not promoted.

It became increasingly apparent that a change in child care practices would not be brought about merely by preparing enthusiastic, well-equipped personnel. Change would entail the creation of a new clinical environment, through the development of the permanent pediatric staff on all levels. This would insure the maintenance of an atmosphere favoring comprehensive care, while supplying at the same time the role models for the teaching of all new and transient personnel.

Although it occurred to me how to affect this change, I did not imagine myself as the agent of change. This came later during the summer of 1966 when I worked for a time as a clinical supervisor in the Pediatric Department of the New York Hospital–Cornell Medical Center, expecting to return to a teaching-consultant position in the fall. Graduate education, in mental health and psychiatric nursing, led to my being called upon frequently during those months to assist in the management of children whose behavior was disruptive. Within a few weeks, the number of referrals so increased that I was devoting my time exclusively to working with this group of patients. As the months passed, the staff came to depend upon this new service for dealing with patients and parents whom they found burdensome. Later, I was asked to join the staff as the mental health consultant for pediatric nursing. In this capacity, I became an insider with the possibility of creating change from within.

The nursing staff made it clear that their need was not so much for consultation on the management of children, but rather for relief from the aggravation that "problem" patients imposed. In their estimation, some children required attention beyond their capacity to supply, and my role was to supply it.

Thus, certain children were singled out for special care by the mental health consultant, while the nursing staff assumed responsibility for their physical welfare. Acting on the principle that one begins wherever permitted, I accepted this direction and worked independently, for several months, with the patients referred to me.

I could have tolerated this arrangement indefinitely for two reasons. First, the deep gratification derived from working in this manner was almost satisfying enough to deter me from the more important goal of motivating active staff involvement in a wider program. Second, I anticipated that a change from a role in which I was accepted conditionally, to a more comprehensive one, would precipitate greater resistance to the work being done.

Indeed, difficulties began when the focus shifted from a crisis orientation approach to a preventive one. The shift was a subtle and painstaking one. It started with keeping the staff informed on patients' progress, even when little interest was demonstrated. In this way, they were introduced to the basic concepts of working with each child. Gradually, a few nurses began to incorporate similar approaches and to parrot behavioral observations and management techniques without recalling the source. This indicated that the process of identification with a new role model had begun. But it was just a start—a long way from true integration of new attitudes and independent functioning. Chapter 1 describes the staff reeducation which leads, subsequently, to an environmental approach to child care.

FROM THE PERSONAL POINT OF VIEW OF THE LIAISON CHILD PSYCHIATRIST

In doing some routine pediatric consultations, I quickly became interested in innovative liaison programs. The flaws in the usual pediatric-psychiatric relationship were the following: calls for consultation from pediatric personnel were mainly for the relief from troublemaking children. Only those psychiatric problems accompanied by gross behavioral manifestations were being noticed. There was usually an emergency atmosphere surrounding the referral, with a potential for friction between members of the respective departments. There was a difference in orientation between the two disciplines, in that pediatric time is in terms of hours, days and weeks, while psychiatric time is in weeks and months. The application of preventive mental health methods was limited to a pilot program in nursing which had been evolving for a year, but was unrecognized by other staff. For the most part, syndromes were allowed to develop rather than being anticipated and modified.

Because their schedules were overloaded, house officers and attending pediatricians were usually interested in having the child dealt with by the psychiatrist and a report made. They applied to psychiatric problems the same attitudes as towards physical or radiation therapy. They were not motivated to acquire diagnostic and therapeutic skills in the area. Therefore, at the outset, the most interested and motivated groups in the area of preventive mental health were the personnel who were most often with the children and who were confronted frequently with the subtle and gross personality characteristics of their charges. These personnel were the nurses, play ladies, school teachers and physical therapists.

It was apparent that to work individually with these groups, however valuable, would be repetitive and would not result in a team approach to the management of children. Representing the largest group and most pivotally situated between the doctors and the other professionals was the nursing mental health consultant. Discussions with her led rapidly to the use of environmental concepts and the inclusion of all people in the hospital that had any relationship to the care of children. Though nursing and psychiatry were applying preventive methods, they were not truly environmental. The latter requires commitment to a total program on the part of each and every discipline that impinges on the child's awareness.

The subsequent large and small conferences that were held on every pediatric floor were open to everyone except parents; and occasionally as professionals relaxed more about their prerogatives, parents also were included. There were many surprises evolving from these "democratic" meetings. Some doctors were reluctant to accept information and formulations from non-doctors. The psychopathology of everyday life was a foreign notion to nearly everyone, as was the application of family and cultural factors to the understanding of individual children. That psychiatry could concern itself with "normal" people was welcomed by some, feared by others. These meetings were the only nonstructured, non-stratified conferences in which persons of different disciplines could speak to each other as equals. This exchange had frequent repercussions; often it was difficult to stay with the topic of one particular child when there were pressing staff conflicts about diagnosis and management, and personal feelings evoked by the patient which needed resolution.

There were obvious built-in strains within pediatric hospital practice. Young doctors who were eager to apply their scientific acumen, and enjoyed their authoritarian position, would often conflict with nurses who had to cope with personal needs in learning to live with great responsibility in carrying out orders and in exercising their maternal ideals. Doctors seemed over-identified with a "magic-bullet" remedy, cure-justifying-any-means attitude. Nurses were identified with the child as victim of illness and of curative procedures in which they often had to inflict pain, without the doctors' ancillary rewards. Play ladies, teachers, nursing aides and attendants were unaccustomed, by years of neglect, to contributing their valuable observations and innovations to the professionals higher on the "status ladder." Thus, some of the people working with children needed "deflation" in their role concept; others needed "inflation" in self-respect and job respect. It came as a new concept that no one could claim exclusive credit for the improvement of the children. The ferment created by the environmental approach pointed out the need for integration of this approach in the education and orientation of all people working with children. Finally, the aim of this philosophy was to go beyond the most advanced prevention methods to so manage the hospitalization experience that it promoted and augmented growth.

1

Reeducation of the Staff for an Environmental Approach

Change in environment is accomplished neither by one person nor by one discipline. For significant change to occur, attention must be directed to influencing the total staff's attitudes on the needs of hospitalized children, and on the policies which determine child care practices.

An environmental approach was not in operation during the early months of our mental health program. The only children who received concentrated attention were those in apparent distress—those who obviously had regressed* or had caused difficulty for the staff. In pediatric literature hospitalization was described as stressful for everyone; but because the number of patients who could be managed by the mental health consultant working independently was limited, only the most disruptive situations were approached.

Expansion of the program to include a greater number of children, and to shift the focus to a preventive approach, required the involvement of the nurses. They held the key positions for determining the environment and experiences to which the children were exposed. In addition, they provided the greatest number of personnel on a 24-hour basis. In an effort to gain their assistance in caring for difficult children, a course in growth and development, and in the management of problems most frequently observed in hospitalized children, was offered. As a result, their ability to detect patients requiring special help increased appreciably, but the situation was only aggravated by the ensuing flood of referrals.

Obviously, other avenues for routine staff involvement had to be found. The nurses' willingness to use a consultant was a first step. However, in order to reach the numbers of children and families needing

---

* Regression is a return to an earlier developmental state, such as recurrence of bed-wetting, baby talk, thumb-sucking, rocking, whining. The regression can be intractable or easily reversible.

9

help and to influence the philosophy of child care in a lasting way, it was essential to have direct nursing participation. Also, in an environment where the care of patients is the responsibility of many professionals, it was important to plan for eventual widespread acceptance among the various paramedical groups.

Opportunity for expansion of the program to include all patients on a preventive basis came through an incident involving Paul, a 5-year-old, who had experienced several previous encounters with hospitalization and surgery, on each occasion becoming more difficult to manage. His reputation preceded him, and anticipation of his arrival caused some consternation. On his last admission for the correction of a bladder-neck obstruction and reimplantation of a ureter, his postoperative behavior was characteristic. He managed to pull out intravenous infusions, tugged at his urinary drainage tubes, regurgitated medications and resorted to frequent tantrums. The separation anxiety he demonstrated was typical of a toddler. Soon after his mother decided that she could safely leave him for a short time, there was a request for help in managing him. His reaction was chaotic; he lashed out at the harassed nurse who tried to distract him, and he banged at the elevator door. The staff was eager to abdicate responsibility for him.

Initially, the approach used to gain this boy's cooperation was commiseration rather than distraction. We encouraged him to recount his problem, to express his feelings regarding his mother's "abandonment" of him (agreeing that it was difficult for him to bear), to talk about his mother— why she left, where she was and how long she would be there; we offered to stay with him in her place until she returned. Our efforts were geared to assuring him that his feelings were understood and were important to us. He became calm and talked about his family, home, friends and interests not connected with hospitalization. Before long, he appeared content with his newly found relationships.

The fact that Paul was beginning to respond to this approach was evident soon after, when he announced the need to urinate. First, we tried to get his impression of what had happened to him, but he remained silent. The importance of helping the child to express his fantasies of his experiences was repeatedly expressed to the staff. This gives the child an opportunity to gain ego mastery over a problem area by putting words to thoughts and provides the occasion to clarify reality. In Paul's case, the confusion was apparent, although he was not able to speak about it directly. He had been told on other occasions the purpose of the drainage tubes, but it did not seem to affect his understanding. This time an explanation was delivered visually. A body outline was sketched including the genitourinary system. This was followed by a simple interpretation of the anatomy and physiology, the congenital defects, surgical correction and the placement and purpose of the tubes; and most significantly in his case, we dealt with the mutilation and castration fantasies common to Paul's period of development. "In the phallic phase . . . whatever part of the body is operated on will take over by displacement the role of the injured genital part."[1] This was done by playful repetition to clarify his understanding in this way: "This is where your operation is, right here on your belly. No other part of your body was operated upon." (Then, pointing to body parts) ". . . not your head, not your ears, not your eyes, nor your nose and mouth, not your arms and chest, not your 'peepee,' nor your legs, feet or toes."

In conjunction with this explanation, Paul was given a stuffed doll on which he was helped to place tubes and bandages in the appropriate areas for his type of surgery. Subsequently with this doll he was helped to pretend administering medication (oral and intramuscular) and to perform the other procedures which were a part of his treatment.

Paul's reaction was striking; he became cooperative with treatments, accepted the staff and was interested in play. This behavioral change became the subject of a nursing team conference the following day. The consensus was that some of Paul's difficulties had been the result of previous hospital trauma, and that much of his turmoil could have been prevented had the new approach been introduced at his first admission. Then the nurses suggested that every patient could profit from similar management by the nursing staff; i.e., of rationalizing treatment to a child, providing human closeness and talking to him about experiences as a way of coping with fear. This was the natural opening which promoted active staff involvement and marked the beginning of change in child care activities on a large scale throughout the department.

Once the nurses themselves suggested how they could contribute, and interest was high, it was important to initiate a program quickly. A series of conferences was held to determine how to proceed. At first because of their experience with Paul, attention was directed primarily to preparing children for urologic surgery, focusing on the special needs and considerations for teaching a specific age group—the child's intellectual and emotional development, the child's fantasies and preoccupations and the kinds of explanations needed for a particular medical or surgical problem. Initially, the number of patients and the type of problems considered were deliberately limited in order to allow time for the development of expertise and gratification.

Each newly admitted patient became the responsibility of one nurse whose work schedule permitted her to care for him on several consecutive days and to become well acquainted with him. In preparation for this assignment, each participant witnessed the procedure the child was to undergo and made an outline of the routine. She then received assistance in introducing and interpreting the material to the child.

The direct supervision and support of nurses during their initial efforts proved effective in diminishing the anxiety they experienced in dealing with negative feelings and fantasy material (related to abandonment, mutilation and death). The meaning of illness to children and their various responses to threats of hospitalization were the topics of numerous group and individual conferences. Understanding in these areas increased the staff's tolerance for difficult behavior, helped them to maintain objectivity and taught them not to assume that children easily accepted treatment.

After the nurses felt comfortable with this approach they allowed parents to witness and to participate in the actual sessions (see Chapter 4). As the staff became more accomplished and satisfied with their progress, they extended their program to include a variety of genitourinary problems. Within a month, news of the work traveled, and requests were received from a few attending physicians and nurses on other units for help in preparing children for many different surgical procedures.

It was easier at this point to conduct continuous orientation classes for the entire department. Included in these sessions were personnel from the x-ray department, intensive care unit, operating and recovery rooms —areas where we needed support and cooperation in order to continue our close relationships with children. Close clinical supervision of new participants was still feasible because it was possible to draw from the more experienced staff for assistance. On occasion the teaching was carried out with medical students, pediatricians, surgeons and recreational therapists who expressed interest. However, because the nursing group was in the best position to offer this aspect of the program consistently, it remained in their purview.

Initially, the program was underplayed. There was never an intent to include experiences which children did not actually witness; for example, no details of the operating room and of the operative procedure were included. Quite often, information on suctioning, endotracheal tubes and monitoring equipment was excluded because the material was too provocative. Unfortunately, the subjects deleted became the preoccupations of our patients. When children were asked to tell, write or draw about their experiences, the themes frequently concerned the unexplained areas and their fears, confusion or anger over being deceived. Clearly, we were not helping children by protecting them from the inevitable. Any omission of information meant leaving them to bear the complete burden. This indicated that the events needed to be presented in an attenuated form, so that they could be viewed with less anxiety, imminence and surprise.

Some of the children were so frightened that they either could not respond immediately to teaching or rejected it altogether. This was primarily true for those who had not received advance preparation by their parents for admission. The prospect of remaining in the hospital was already sufficiently alarming. For them, a more successful introduction was to talk about the many other children that were also in the hospital—their reasons for admission, their treatment and the equipment used in their care. Thus, it was possible to touch upon the relevant areas indirectly. In addition, much of the essential information was given through playing out procedures on dolls, by allowing the children to take the roles of physicians and nurses—caretakers instead of victims.

One of the major difficulties was in finding the time for work with the child prior to the scheduled procedure. For minor treatment (from a medical, not the child's point of view), the essential aspects of the procedure could be covered even when a child was admitted the afternoon before the event. There was not adequate time, however, for adjustment to the hospital or for thinking through and asking questions about the information given. In complicated procedures, such as cardiac surgery, the material could not be delivered in a condensed fashion, because too much, too quickly, would be overwhelming for the patients. Because the children also required intensive physical preparation, competition from physicians and technicians from various departments—x-ray, hematology and cardiology—was great. Therefore it was necessary to interpret to pediatricians and surgeons, the importance of adequate time for preparation and to gain their cooperation in admitting patients earlier.

After several revisions and trials, a manual of guidelines for teaching children of all ages was produced; with specific instructions on—approaching various age groups, when to begin teaching, the content to be covered, the amount of information recommended for one session, and actual explanations and terminology for each procedure.

As the program developed, we adopted a set of attractive body outlines, and produced a number of tools which enhanced our efforts. Patient dolls (male and female, attired in johnny shirts) were made for us by the Volunteer Department and models of frequently used equipment were constructed (see Chapter 6).

During the first year, the greatest progress in reeducating the staff was made in several areas offering the least resistance. Initially the distribution of time and energy was unequal, and deliberately so. Those areas where personnel were uninterested or antagonistic were temporarily avoided. However, the passage of time and staff turnover (a mixed blessing) eventually opened up floors formerly not amenable to change.

Some of the staff complained that their patients had been neglected by the mental health team, an excellent sign of their readiness for the program. When this occurred, it was because the nurses were already motivated by the conviction that the new approach was important. Consequently, this attitude contributed greatly to their successful participation. A number of our nurses stated that they were encouraged through observing the success of colleagues in working with children. They were impressed by the actual demonstration of techniques and the discussion of principles involved. As students, they had heard repeatedly how important it was to support children and their families and to help them cope with the difficult experiences; however, they had not been taught how to do it, nor did they see it being done.

Others were convinced by the excellent results, which were common occurrences, consistently achieved. The children showed greater acceptance of staff members, ability to participate in treatments and ease in expressing their feelings. There was less preoccupation with procedures and illness, a greater capacity for socialization, and interest in play and tolerance for reasonable periods of separation from parents. The adjustment process for patients who were admitted repeatedly for chronic illnesses became easier because they had already mastered many of the fears hospitalization presented.

RESISTANCE

It would have been amazing had the program developed without opposition. Resistance occurred in many forms. At the outset, as long as the mental health consultant worked independently, there was little objection. Of course, there were a few who commented disparagingly on the need for a mental health service, but this was offset, for the most part, by those who were genuinely pleased to have assistance with patients. More overt resentment was demonstrated when tentative demands were made on the nursing staff for direct participation in the management of children with behavior problems. Resentment also occurred in response to the suggestion that many of the regressive behavior and disciplinary problems could be eliminated or modified by staff members themselves. The most common response to this was defensiveness—how could nurses be expected to carry out such functions when the pressures of work were already great?

Though they were never coerced into assuming roles which they did not want, efforts were made to influence acceptance indirectly. However, a few of the nurses could not tolerate the discomfort they felt in witnessing the new approach, even though they were not actively engaged in it. Consequently, they resigned. This was balanced, fortunately, by those who were attracted by the program and joined the staff specifically for learning new skills in pediatric care.

Several children with whom the mental health consultant was working were the focus of early resistance. One instance concerned 9-year-old Mario admitted for multiple operations to correct facial deformities. Prior to admission and during early hospitalization, he manifested severe emotional disturbance. He was referred for special attention because he was unmanageable, and physically and socially repulsive to most people. During a 5-month period, it was possible to win his trust and help him modify his behavior toward more acceptable standards. In comparison to previous behavior, he now developed remarkable control of violence and acquired the ability to verbalize his feelings and to postpone immediate pleasure. His change brought with it unfortunate repercussions. Whereas originally the plan for working with this child during the most trying periods won the full support of the medical and nursing staff, his improvement brought open resistance. Changes in his management were ordered without prior discussion. Those features and activities which were supportive in his care were suddenly eliminated. In addition he was subjected to various provocative incidents which served to break down newly established controls.

The situation was analogous to that of resistance on the part of family members to a patient's progress in therapy—hospital personnel, in this instance, taking on the roles of family members. The staff was reluctant to accept the change evident in Mario. For some time, he had been a useful scapegoat; and as is the case frequently in the treatment of a disturbed child, the family was unwilling to give up the gratification they derived from the child's negative behavior. One often sees parents attempting to devaluate the therapist or change agent by opposing his efforts. A similar attitude on the part of the staff was also evident toward the mental health consultant.

In Mario's case it was possible to work around the situation by enlisting the support of staff members who understood the dynamics and were willing to share in the responsibility for his care. In other cases, however, when support was not forthcoming, it was necessary to abandon work with the children rather than to increase the resistance of the staff, stress to the child or to place the program in greater jeopardy. (See the story of Kate, page 231.)

The most serious resistance developed with the medical staff. In the early phases, no organized effort was made to include them in the program except on an administrative level. It was hoped that enough support would develop among the nursing group to be influential in gaining their support and that a psychiatrist would eventually introduce the program. This strategy produced the desired results. Whenever derogatory comments were made to the nurses about their "frivolous" work or about the mental health consultant's interference in medical care, the program and services were asserted to be integral to comprehensive care and not contrary to medical goals. By the time opposition grew, there were already small numbers of nurses, attending physicians and resident pediatricians who could defend the program. They were quick to grasp how the innovations could serve to support children and parents during periods of crises.

However, long after preventive mental health principles had been introduced into the program, more serious resistance was still to come. It began in full force as the program, once again, underwent a shift in focus—from a preventive to an environmental approach. With the introduction of the liaison psychiatrist, multidisciplinary patient-centered conferences were instituted; and as a result, divergent points of view and basic difficulties in working relationships were exposed.

Over a period of months, contrary to traditional role expectations, the nurses emerged as confident, knowledgeable and vocal participants. They lost their usual reticence in offering ideas and were proud to claim results and credit for their work. This view was shared by the parents, who gave the nurses enthusiastic praise when discussing their children with the medical staff.

Tension grew among a small but militant group of resident physicians who refused to acknowledge the nurses' expanded role in the psychosocial aspects of patient care. They accused the nurses of "taking over"—of resisting the physicians' leadership. Those nurses who also resisted change encouraged them in this point of view. Together, they were instrumental in convincing a number of pediatricians, who had formerly accepted the program, to withdraw their support. This phase of resistance was most damaging as it affected the treatment of several patients who were currently the subjects of controversy (see the stories of Calton and Michael, Chapter 8), polarized groups and weakened the influence of the nascent mental health team consisting of the mental health nurse and the liaison psychiatrist.

The neglected area of pediatrics had begun to look appealing, once techniques were developed that obviously worked. However, physicians saw the contributions of others to patient management as a loss of control over medical care; and they saw the increasing appreciation of psychosocial factors as a devaluation of their work in physical treatment. They then sought to discredit the mental health leadership and thereby to minimize the importance of the area in which they felt threatened.

The mental health team realized that they were working in an institution, similar to many, in which innovators are seen as people trying to gain power at the expense of others. They realized, too, that a change in the behavior of one discipline (nursing) was bound to affect its relationship to any closely allied group—just as treatment of one member brings about counteraction in the total family.

There was a danger that the discord in relationships, as a result of the nurses' professional growth, would bring about the dissolution of the program; nevertheless, forces were working for it. Both nursing and medical administration gave support. A number of pediatricians convinced their reluctant colleagues of the integral contributions of paramedical personnel to comprehensive care. Furthermore, the nurses banded together to reaffirm their belief in the program and to insist on its continuation.

Although the program is now operating, its acceptance cannot be taken for granted. Until professionals are prepared in their basic education to think about total child care, the environmental approach will have to fight continually for survival. Paradoxically, it is most endangered when it succeeds, as this incurs envy and fear leading to resistance.

REFERENCE

1. Freud, A.: The role of bodily illness in the mental life of children. *In* Eissler, R., *et al.* (eds.): The Psychoanalytic Study of the Child. vol. 7, pp. 74-75, New York, International Universities Press, 1952.

BIBLIOGRAPHY

Bates, B.: Doctor and nurse: changing roles and relations. New Eng. J. Med., *283*:129, 1970.

Finch, S. M., and McDermott, J. F., Jr.: Psychiatry for the Pediatrician. New York, W. W. Norton, 1970.

Foley, J. M.: Some psychological aspects of hospitalization. *In* Schulman, J.: Management of Emotional Disorders in Pediatric Practice. Chicago, Yearbook Medical Publishers, 1967.

Geist, H.: A Child Goes to the Hospital. Springfield, Ill., Charles C Thomas, 1965.

Georgopoulos, B. S., and Christman, L.: The clinical nurse specialist: a role model. Amer. J. Nurs., *70*:1030, 1970.

Gordon, M.: The clinical specialist as a change agent. Nurs. Outlook, *17*:37, 1969.

Jessner, L., *et al.*: Emotional implications of tonsillectomy and adenoidectomy on children. *In* Eissler, R., *et al.* (eds.): The Psychoanalytic Study of the Child. vol. 7. New York, International Universities Press, 1952.

Johnson, D. E., Wilcox, J. A., and Moidel, H. C.: The clinical specialist as a practitioner. Amer. J. Nurs., *67*:2298, 1967.

Langford, W. S.: The child in the pediatric hospital: adaptation to illness and hospitalization. Amer. J. Orthopsychiat., *31*:667, 1961.

Petrillo, M.: Preventing hospital trauma in pediatric patients. Amer. J. Nurs., *68*:1468, 1968.

Prugh, D. G., *et al.*: A study of the emotional reactions of children and families to hospitalization and illness. Amer. J. Orthopsychiat., *23*:70, 1953.

Shore, M. F., Geiser, R. L., Wolman, H. M.: Constructive uses of a hospital experience. Children, *12*:3, 1965.

Vernon, D. T., *et al.*: The Psychological Responses of Children to Hospitalization and Illness: A Review of the Literature. Springfield, Ill., Charles C Thomas, 1965.

2

A Working Knowledge of Childhood

The challenge of caring for children is to combine a sensitive awareness of the individual child with an awareness of all the valuable diverse facts and theories of the past 75 years in order to achieve a synthesis that could be called a developmental adaptive assessment.

One cannot know everything there is to know about a child. Observation, history and interview supply only a portion of the picture; this is the raw data. It is possible to arrive at a more comprehensive and complete "profile" of an individual, when data are interpreted in the context of experience and theoretical knowledge.

General knowledge works in two ways: It tells us what to look for, and it helps us to make sense of what we find. The various theories of this chapter added to clinical experiences gathered over time will lead to a structured general knowledge needed by professionals. Unorganized experience, however fascinating, can lead to chaos. Knowledge of theories alone can become dull and empty. When combined, there is the greatest possibility for creative and progressive evaluation of children.

In later chapters this combination will be seen to be one of the basic components that influences this innovative, environmental plan for each child.

In the following pages, many of the important theories of growth and development are outlined. Presented are the beginnings for a basic, organized approach to children at different ages. The bibliography contains the most recent reviews and writings of these theorists. However, no summary can do justice to the rich clinical and theoretical material that would reward the reader who goes beyond this chapter.

THE FIRST YEAR

DEVELOPMENTAL LANDMARKS CENTRAL NERVOUS SYSTEM MATURATION (Gesell)	INTERACTIONAL, FIELD AND SYSTEMS THEORIES (Spitz, Escalona, Sander)	STAGES OF INTELLECTUAL DEVELOPMENT (Piaget)
1 day to 1 month: Responds to bell; makes crawling movements	When baby sends a cue to mother (cry of distress), how appropriate is her response? This is also called the degree of fit between mother and child.	Sensorimotor stage from birth to 2 years:
1 month: Follows an object to midline; coos, gurgles, makes a fist; shows tonic neck reflex	Development of mutual regulatory and reciprocal interchanges between mother and child; e.g., synchrony of sleeping, eating, elimination—between mother and baby.	"Neonatal reflex" substage: complete self-world undifferentiation
2 months: Social smile; 180° visual pursuit; transitory reflexes—Moro, suck, grasp		"Primary circular" substage: simple acts are repeated
4 months: Reaches for objects	In the first few months, the baby gradually takes more of the initiative in signalling his needs.	"Secondary circular" substage: there is repetition of acts that affect an object
5 months: Rolls over		
6–8 months: Raking grasp; sitting, crawling		
9 months: Crude purposeful release of objects grasped	With time there is an increased intensity in the baby's expression of needs.	"Secondary circular" substage: actions become committed to memory
10 months: Pincer grasp		
10–14 months: Walks; knows 3 to 4 words		

THE FIRST YEAR

PSYCHOSOCIAL TASKS OR CRISES
(Erikson)

Trust or mistrust: The first year encompasses the time when confidence in having needs met and in feeling physically safe takes place. When needs are consistently met, anticipation of satisfaction occurs. The result is optimism. When a child anticipates frustration, pessimism about the world develops.

INDIVIDUAL DIFFERENCES
(Chess)

By 3 months it is possible to determine differences in activity and temperament which remain the same for the next few years.

The 9 differences are:
- Active/passive
- Regular/irregular rhythmicity
- Intensity of movement (high/low)
- Approach/withdraw
- Adaptation/nonadaptation
- High/low response to stimulus
- Positive/negative mood
- High/low selectivity, attention span, persistence
- High/low distractability

Certain combinations are bad; e.g., if passive, high intensity or withdrawal and nonadaptation. Other combinations are good; e.g., if mood is positive, adaptation high, and strong approach.

PSYCHOSEXUAL STAGES
(Sigmund Freud)

Infant wants the mother and fears her loss lest body needs go unsatisfied and create increased tension. Mother gives satisfaction and relieves tension. From birth to 18 months is the ORAL stage. This includes respiratory, sensory, and kinesthetic responses. The mode of relationship is incorporative. With a good mother, baby's energies gradually decrease in concentration on the self and increasingly are directed toward the mother. The threat of losing the mother produces increased tension in the infant who is left without the object (mother) on whom he has placed all his energies. This is primary anxiety. Defenses that the infant and toddler use to cope with anxiety are imitation, avoidance and denial.

THE FIRST YEAR

EGO PSYCHOLOGY
(Anna Freud et al.)

0–3 months: Normal autism: Complete self-absorbing without awareness of the world

4–18 months: Symbiotic phase (Mahler); mother seen as an extension of child's body and needs (and vice versa)

6–10 months: Stranger anxiety begins; shows that infant can distinguish between the symbiotic object (mother) and all others

8–24 months: Separation anxiety: Reluctant to lose sight of mother; beginnings of transitional objects (Winnicott)—partly representing mother, partly the self (e.g., an animal or security blanket)

EGO/INSTINCT ACCOMMODATION-DEVELOPMENTAL LINES
(Anna Freud)

A. From dependency to emotional self-reliance and adult relationships:

In the first year, there is a biologic unit with mother. This symbiosis then evolves toward separation and individuation.

B. From body dependency toward body independence:

1. May have difficulties in feeding and in achieving synchrony with the mother; e.g., oral deprivation may be consequent to abrupt weaning, with rejection of new tastes in foods. By the end of the first year, child begins to feed himself.

2. Has complete freedom from bladder and bowel control.

3. Has no responsibility in body management—the mother does everything. Positive feeling towards his own body protects the infant from self-damage.

4. Infant is totally egocentric (selfish or narcissistic). Other persons are a disturbance of the relationship to mother and are treated as lifeless objects

5. Infant's own body is the source of orientation and play; e.g., interest in mouth and skin sensation of self and mother. Transitional object begins at this time.

ONE YEAR TO THREE-AND-A-HALF YEARS

DEVELOPMENTAL LANDMARKS CENTRAL NERVOUS SYSTEM MATURATION (Gesell)	INTERACTIONAL FIELD AND SYSTEMS THEORIES (Bowlby, Lorenz)	STAGES OF INTELLECTUAL DEVELOPMENT (Piaget)
1½ years: 2 cube tower; scribbles with crayon; knows ten words; capable of bowel training	From birth to age 2, the mother is the central integrator of attachment behavior. Social releasers from baby such as sucking, crying, following, clinging, smiling—all lead to behavior responses in the mother. Stranger anxiety at 24 months coincides with the height of this adaptation to the mother. Aggression is the opposite to attachment and needs discouragement, not punishment. Aggression is heightened by mother's teaching this to the child, or by forced weaning.	2 years: By this time the child performs mental combinations by trial and error. There is relatively coherent organization of sensorimotor action. The child learns that certain actions have a specific effect on the environment. There is beginning symbolic activity. There is recognition of constancy of external objects. The world is represented primitively. Symbols and figures stand for objects. Egocentric thinking predominates. (The child refers every event to himself; e.g., if mother leaves, it is due to his action.)
2 years: 6 cube tower		
2½ years: Three-word sentences; names 6 body parts; pronouns		
3 years: Tricycle; copies O; matches four colors		
3½ years: Talks to self and others; takes turns; walks on a line		

ONE YEAR TO THREE-AND-A-HALF YEARS

PSYCHOSOCIAL TASKS OR CRISES
(Erikson)

By the age of 3½, there is established on the basis of previous adaption a general attitude of initiative illustrated by—"I am what I imagine I can be." Each effort is preceded by fantasy play. Failure at this stage is shown by guilty reluctance to explore, by doubt, by sense of uselessness.

PSYCHOSEXUAL STAGES
(Sigmund Freud)

One-and-a-half to 3½ years is the anal and urethral stage when elimination and retention are the modes. Muscles are used to express control and inhibition. Feelings are displaced onto objects or symbols and projected onto others; e.g., "If I feel this way, others must also."

EGO PSYCHOLOGY
(Anna Freud et al.)

From 12 to 28 months the infant and toddler are in the separation-individuation phase (Mahler). This is seen in self-feeding from 17 to 30 months. This is the height of the oppositional syndrome (assertiveness to begin differentiation of the child from the mother [Levy]).

From 2 to 3, there is messiness, exploration, parallel play, pleasure in looking and being looked at. At approximately 3, a self-concept begins. Early conscience occurs—by way of identification with parents. Orderliness, disgust, masturbation and curiosity are expressions of instinct development. There is also cooperative play, fantasy play and imaginary playmates based on magical-thinking (that things happen when they are wished).

ONE YEAR TO THREE-AND-A-HALF YEARS

EGO/INSTINCT ACCOMMODATION-DEVELOPMENTAL LINES
(Anna Freud)

A. In second to fourth year, the mother is a part-object, or an instrument, who captures the child's interest because of his needs. By the third year, the child has a constant mental representation of the mother regardless of her absence or lack of gratification. The child acts as if he remembers, misses her, and doubts that she will return. Toward the end of the third year, the ambivalent (anal-preoedipal) stage is exemplified by love alternating with hate, clinging with defiance.

B. In developing toward body independence:

1. Though there is self-feeding, food is the battle-ground in differentiation from mother—("battle for the spoon"-Levy). There is a craving for sweets, food fads and food refusal which is always aimed at mother.

2. Body products become invested with sexual and aggressive energy. There are swings between love and hate, curiosity and neglect, emptying and hoarding. The instinctual drives in going from the oral to the anal zone lead to increasing oppositional behavior (stubbornness).

3. With increasing ego functioning and awareness of cause and effect, the body is protected and dangerous wishes are controlled under the reality principle; e.g., fire, heights, water are facts which must be respected.

4. From 1 to 3½, the toddler sees other persons as helpers in carrying out his wishes. By 4 years they become partners and objects in their own right—to be feared and admired. At the same time, earliest friend-ships begin.

5. In progressing from interest solely in his own body and in play, the toddler changes from one specific transi-tional object to other inanimate objects which are treated with love, hate and invested with sexual and aggressive energy. By the middle of the third year, cuddly toys fade out except at night. Play helps direct drive energies to socially useful pursuits.

THREE-AND-A-HALF TO SIX-AND-A-HALF YEARS (PRESCHOOL)

DEVELOPMENTAL LANDMARKS
(Gesell)

4 years: Copies X; throws overhand; develops early right/left orientation

4½ years: Copies □

5 years: Copies △; ties knots in string

6 years: Prints name; ties shoes; makes single function similarities; rides two wheeler; copies ◇

STAGES OF INTELLECTUAL DEVELOPMENT
(Piaget)

Between 3 and 7 is the stage called "preoperational" or "preconceptual." Thought is intuitive, prelogical (magical). There begins the first relatively unorganized and fumbling attempts to grasp the new and strange world of symbols. Thinking is still egocentric—conclusions are based on feelings or on what the child would like to believe.

PSYCHOSEXUAL STAGE
(Sigmund Freud)

Four years old—the phallic stage (locomotor). Intrusive and inclusive modes —there is much interest in competence, prowess and dominance. Oedipal is the last phase. The child in this phase likes the parent of the opposite sex and tends to turn away from the parent of the same sex. There is a fear of castration by the parent of the same sex. This leads to repression of original oedipal wishes. Ambivalence occurs toward both parents. The resolution is the renunciation of the heterosexual incestuous object, and later a search to find someone like the parent of the opposite sex. (Normally occurs after age 6.)

THREE-AND-A-HALF TO SIX-AND-A-HALF YEARS (PRESCHOOL)

EGO PSYCHOLOGY
(Anna Freud)

4 years: Mastery is most important as shown by task completion; magical-thinking decreases; rivalry with parent of same sex continues

5 years: Follows rules; pre-latency type play gives way to latency play in which skills count

6 years: Shows problem solving achievements, voluntary hygiene, competition, hobbies and ritualistic play

EGO/INSTINCT ACCOMMODATION-DEVELOPMENT LINES
(Anna Freud)

A. The phallic period (4 to 5 years):

Closer to true mutual relationships, though still wishes for exclusive rights with each parent. Castration anxiety at its height, also exhibitionism.

B. In developing toward body independence:

1. 4½ to 6½—food representing mother, fades out, though food retains a magical quality; i.e., overeating leads to getting fat and having a baby. Eating can become sexualized (anorexia). It may become involved in reaction formation; i.e., food refusal is a way of denying wish to devour the mother.

2. By 5, attitudes toward bowel and bladder control come to resemble mother's through identification and ego-superego maturation. Ego develops inner defenses against urethral and anal wishes (total freedom to mess) which now get channelled into such patterns as punctuality, neatness and miserliness.

[28]

SIX-AND-A-HALF TO ELEVEN YEARS (SCHOOL AGE)

DEVELOPMENTAL LANDMARKS
(Gesell)

7 years: Makes simple opposite analogies; knows days of the week

8 years: Counts 5 digits forward; defines *brave* and *nonsense*

9 years: Knows seasons, rhymes

10 years: Counts 4 digits reversed; expresses and defines *pity, grief* and *surprise*

STAGES OF INTELLECTUAL DEVELOPMENT
(Piaget)

Seven to 12 years is the stage of "Concrete Operational Thought." Conceptual organization takes on stability and coherence. There are rational, well-organized adaptations. Conceptual framework is brought to bear on objects in world. Physical qualities are seen as constant despite change in size, shape, weight and volume.

PSYCHOSOCIAL TASKS OR CRISES
(Erikson)

Between 6 and 11, the child's skills and values expand to include those of the neighborhood and school. Successful adaptations here lead to industry (I am what I learn); unsuccessful to inferiority.

SIX-AND-A-HALF TO ELEVEN YEARS (SCHOOL AGE)

PSYCHOSEXUAL STAGES
(Sigmund Freud)

Latency occurs between 7 and 11 years. The sexual drive is controlled and repressed. There is use of the unconscious mechanisms of isolation (separation of an idea from its accompanying feeling), pseudocompulsion (repeated rituals and mannerisms as foot tapping, hair pulling, avoiding stepping on cracks), turning to the opposite (a child will deny her hatred of the new sibling by saying she loves him), and sublimation of instinctual wishes (channelling of drives into socially acceptable outlets; e.g., oral needs may evolve into gourmet interests). Emphasis during latency is also on development of skills and talents.

EGO PSYCHOLOGY
(Anna Freud)

The 9-year-old is: Rational about food; companionable; invested in non-family relationships

Autonomous ego functions develop—automatically behaves in areas that formerly created conflict; e.g., uses words instead of violence, comfortably obeys most rules, can postpone immediate gratification

EGO/INSTINCT ACCOMMODATION-DEVELOPMENTAL LINES
(Anna Freud)

A. In relationships:

The 6- to 11-year-old transfers interest to others outside the family. This and the normal disillusionment with parents leads to the feeling of having been adopted (the "family romance" where an idealized set of parents is envisioned).

B. In developing toward body independence:

1. There is the final phasing out of the sexualization of eating with a rational attitude.

2. In bowel and bladder control, cleanliness becomes disconnected from object ties and becomes an autonomous ego-superego concern.

3. Body management completely taken over by child.

ELEVEN TO EIGHTEEN YEARS (ADOLESCENCE)

DEVELOPMENTAL LANDMARKS (Gesell)	STAGES OF INTELLECTUAL DEVELOPMENT (Piaget)
11 years on: Knows where sun sets, about a microscope, nitrogen, why oil floats. Divides 74 by 4, makes abstract similarities, understands C.O.D. Repeats 6 digits forward; 5 reverse.	Twelve years—formal operational thought: Deals effectively with reality and also with abstract propositional statements and the world of possibility. Cognition is adult type. Deductive reasoning developed. Can evaluate logic and quality of own thinking. Increase in abstract powers leads to capacity to deal with laws and principles. Still egocentric at times. Important ideals and attitudes develop in late adolescence and early adulthood.

Summary of Piaget

Overall: Adaptation and coping change and reorganize the mind. Complex stimulation in a favorable environment causes accommodation of mental structures to the nuances of reality.

All mental function derives from motor actions on objects. Growth of intelligence is based on the transformation of these motor patterns into thought. Incorporation of the novel is assimilation; reorganization of past thoughts and memories to more closely approximate the assimilated novelty is accommodation. Development is the interplay between assimilation and accommodation. When accommodation stops with respect to an assimilation, then behavior is adapted or a balance then exists between assimilation and accommodation. It is a human tendency to assimilate all possible novelty. It is novelty that motivates repetition or circular reactions in order to give more contact and exposure to the unfamiliar.

ELEVEN TO EIGHTEEN YEARS (ADOLESCENCE)

PSYCHOSOCIAL TASKS OR CRISES
(Erikson)

Between 12 and 17, the youth seeks to "know what I am." The predominant values are those of adolescent peer group and leadership. Identity is the outcome. If the individual is unsuccessful, there is "identity diffusion."

After 17, ability to love is paramount with success being shown by intimacy. Lack of success leads to isolation and alienation. Values at this time: fidelity, friendship, and cooperation. Sexual behavior and competition approach the adult type.

PSYCHOSEXUAL STAGES
(Sigmund Freud)

Eleven to 13 years (Puberty): Importance of peer group, recapitulation of oedipal struggle consequent to resurgence of sexual drives. Contact with the opposite sex is once more seen as potentially dangerous as it leads to competition with others of the same sex and possible defeat. In addition, seeking a new idealized self to replace the parents who are now discredited, often causes attraction to another of the same sex who has admirable qualities ("normal" homosexual phase).

Thirteen to 18 years: Adolescent-adult modes of leadership. Coping mechanisms are intellectualization, rationalization, asceticism.

Genitality achieved with the primacy of heterosexual orgasm. Ability to love and work are the culmination of these stages.

EGO PSYCHOLOGY
(Anna Freud)

Adolescent revolt loosens ties to family. Cliques develop with friends. Responsibility and independent work habits solidify.

Late adolescence: Heterosexual interests lead to marriage and parental readiness. Recreational and intellectual activities prepare the young adult for vocational choice and later commitment.

ELEVEN TO EIGHTEEN YEARS (ADOLESCENCE)

EGO/INSTINCT ACCOMMODATION-
DEVELOPMENTAL LINES
(Anna Freud)

A. In relationships and self-reliance:

Eleven- to 13-year-old preadolescents have a return of ambivalence and weakening of phallic and latency accomplishments.

Thirteen- to 15-year-old adolescents loosen ties to parents.

Fifteen years on: Genital supremacy. There is an active, healthy struggle to finally control the impulses of the first 6 years. Relationships acquire give and take qualities—mutual self-help.

B. All development lines toward body independence continue to solidify. During adolescence there is a final voluntary indorsement of the rules of hygiene and medical necessities. The ability to work is the culmination of the developmental line which began with play, task completion, and the use of inanimate objects. Control of destructive impulses, frustration tolerance, and living by the reality principle (future gratifications may involve short term renunciations) are also necessary for adult work.

COMMENT ON ANNA FREUD'S
DEVELOPMENTAL LINES

Each of the Lines A, B1, B2, B3, B4, B5 represent an intrapsychic balance between ego-superego, and the id. No one of these 6 Lines is to be used exclusively in assessing a child. It is more of a clustering or profile of different intrapsychic dynamics which gives the true picture. Thus a 14-year-old boy could have several close friends, be overeating, be sloppy, brush his teeth, practice body building, have several hobbies, and be doing mediocre work in school. He would have attained different stages in his separate developmental lines. From this data, the conclusion is drawn that he just approaches emotional adolescence.

BIBLIOGRAPHY

Blos, P.: The Young Adolescent, Clinical Studies. New York, The Free Press, 1970.

Chess, S.: Psychiatric disorders of childhood: healthy responses, developmental disturbances, and stress or reactive disorders, Part I: Infancy and childhood. *In* Freedman, A. M., and Kaplan, H. T.: Comprehensive Textbook of Psychiatry. Baltimore, Williams & Wilkins, 1967.

Erikson, E. H.: Childhood and Society. ed. 2, pp. 247-274, New York, W. W. Norton, 1963.

————: Identity: Youth and Crisis. New York, W. W. Norton, 1968.

Freud, A.: The Psychoanalytical Treatment of Children. New York, International Universities Press, 1965.

————: The Ego and the Mechanisms of Defense. rev. ed. New York, International Universities Press, 1966.

————: Normality and Pathology in Childhood: Assessments of Development. New York, International Universities Press, 1965.

Gesell, A.: The First Five Years of Life. New York, Harper & Row, 1940.

————: The Child from Five to Ten. New York, Harper & Row, 1946.

Gesell, A., *et al.:* Youth: The Years from Ten to Sixteen. New York, Harper & Row, 1956.

Hall, C. S.: A Primer of Freudian Psychology. New York, World Publishing Company, 1954.

Hollitscher, W.: Sigmund Freud, An Introduction. Freeport, New York, Books for Libraries Press, 1970.

Ilg, F., and Ames, L.: Child Behavior. New York, Harper & Row, 1951.

Josselyn, I. M.: The Happy Child: A Psychoanalytic Guide to Emotional and Social Growth. New York, Random House, 1955.

Levy, D. M.: Oppositional syndromes and oppositional behavior. *In* Hoch, P., and Zubin, J. (eds.): Psycho-pathology of Childhood. vol. X. New York, Grune & Stratton, 1955.

Lidz, T.: The Person: His Development Throughout the Life Cycle. New York, Basic Books, 1968.

Lorenz, K.: On Aggression. New York, Harcourt Brace Jovanovich, 1966.

Mahler, M. S., and Furer, M. S.: On Human Symbiosis and Vicissitudes of Individuation. vol. 1: Infantile Psychoses. New York, International Universities Press, 1968.

Piaget, J., and Inhelder, B.: The Psychology of the Child. New York, Basic Books, 1969.

Report of the Joint Commission on Mental Health: Crisis in Child Mental Health: Challenge for the 1970's. Chap. 8. Social-psychological aspects of normal growth and development: adolescents and youth. New York, Harper & Row, 1969.

Sander, L. W.: Adaptive relationships in early mother-child interaction. J. Amer. Acad. Child Psychiat. *3*:231, 1964.

Solnit, A. J., and Provence, S. A.: Modern Perspectives in Child Development. New York, International Universities Press, 1963.

Spitz, R. A.: The First Year of Life. New York, International Universities Press, 1965.

Thomas, A., *et al.:* The origin of personality. Sci. Amer., *223*:102, 1970.

von Bertalanffy, L.: General system theory and psychiatry. *In* Arieti, S.: American Handbook of Psychiatry. vol. 3. New York, Basic Books, 1966.

Winnicott, D. W.: Collected Papers, Through Pediatrics to Psychoanalysis. pp. 229-242. London, Tavistock Publications, 1958.

Wolff, P. H.: The Developmental Psychologies of Jean Piaget and Psychoanalysis. Psychological Issues, vol. 2, No. 1. New York, International Universities Press, 1960.

————: The role of biological rhythms in early psychological development. Bull. Menninger Clin., *31*:197, 1967.

3

Family Assessment and Management

Discerning the pattern of relationships in a family can be formidable. Interactions are complex; yet, unless the generally expected patterns are compared with the data from a particular family, a preliminary assessment cannot be made. This rough estimate of the current adaptation helps to predict behavior under stress. Such anticipations are valid, since any group will retain its basic characteristics even in crisis.

Cultural

One of the ways to deepen understanding of individuals and families is to have a knowledge of their cultural background. Many families will react to the stress of illness in character with their heritage. These reactions affect the child and also the hospital staff. For instance, Spiegel contrasts the time orientation of the foreign-born Italian working class with middle class Americans.[1] He shows in basic ways how deep the differences can be—the Italians emphasize present, past and future in that order; Americans, the future, present, and past. With this knowledge, professionals would be able to understand the difference between the Italian grandparents, who would be concerned with the origins of an illness, and the Americanized parents, who would consider how the illness affects the child's school work and future. Thus, the professional could expect an already existing conflict between parents and grandparents or between foreign-born parents and staff.

Because of the general American mixture of cultures,[2] there are no cultural patternings that exist in a pure form in America today. Because the differences within cultures are as great as those between them, it is best to rely on socioeconomic style and family development in addition to cultural type in order to make family assessments. However, it is important to avoid stereotyping a family because of its cultural or economic background. This can be accomplished by the nurse and physician if more is learned about the family as individuals. Each family is unique, and generalizations about low income or culturally deprived families serve as a starting point in understanding the problems families face.

Socioeconomic

The atmosphere in low socioeconomic homes is not only conducive to increasing incidence and prevalence of illness, but also to early pervasive impediments to the attainment of school success and sociability. Because of the number of culture-of-poverty people in hospitals and clinics, a thorough knowledge is important. The Report of the Joint Commission on Mental Health of Children[3] outlines much of this information. (See chart, page 44.) The U.S. Government booklet, *Growing Up Poor* shows how all races at the poverty level are affected by the stability or instability of both emotional and economic climate.

Hollingshead and Redlich describe 5 classes of people who are easily defined by residential address, occupation and years of schooling completed by the household head. Each class furthermore has cultural traits that cluster about it and sharpen its definition. These authors further demonstrate the type and prevalence of mental illness that occurs in correlation with class; e.g., character neuroses are found most frequently in the highest classes (1 and 2) while antisocial and immature reactions are found in the lowest class (5).[4]

These distinctions are also true in the physical realm in which the lowest class is found to have the poorest health; e.g., malnutrition, dental caries, obesity, and accidental ingestions (in childhood).

Hospital personnel need to be attuned to their reactions to these particular classes. Hollingshead and Redlich demonstrate that a bias does exist against certain classes in spite of "professional objectivity," which supposedly makes no distinctions. Because professionals come predominantly from classes 2 and 3, they have a natural unfamiliarity with classes 1, 4, and 5, and tend to have overcritical or oversolicitous attitudes toward them.

Family Development

Families differ according to their development as a unit. A young family under 3 years duration, still settling marital roles, is insecure as to what tasks are masculine and feminine, and often tries to ignore outside influences in developing its identity. The couple may turn to professionals as healthier influences than their relatives, who continue to treat them as they did before marriage. Money handling and financial planning are realistic issues. There is always the adjustment between what they expected from marriage and what they are getting. Inexperience with children leads them to anxious overconcern with development and child care practices. They are reluctant to rely on spontaneous feeling.

A family established for 4 to 10 years is less susceptible to outside influence and has routinized patterns of husband-wife roles and parent-child relationships. There is more stability in economic matters and with respect to relatives. The autonomy and independence of the children, and the relationships between the children and to school are new issues. This more established family is not as prone to sudden mood fluctuation as the younger family. In reaction to their earlier overconcern with growth and development, this couple may become so casual as to ignore important factors in the development of their children.

An older established family of 10 to 20 years has set patterns to the direction of their lives. However, they need to learn how to adjust to the difficulties of normal separation and emancipation of their children. These adjustments can be complicated by illness. For example, an adolescent who has been predominantly out of the home and involved with peer group activities, can be quite a problem if he needs once again to be dependent on his parents because of illness.

Family Composition

The size of the family and the child's position in it can alert the professional to certain probabilities. However, generalizations are misleading; e.g., an only child can have regular, intimate companions and a child from a large family can be isolated and lonely. Although a middle child may have neither the advantage of the oldest nor the immunity of the baby, he may, however, avoid the high expectations imposed on a first child and escape the indulgence of the youngest. The youngest child may have to scramble and fight for love and attention, or he may become the spoiled family mascot. A large family may be able to give "each according to his needs" and provide a sense of unity and closeness; yet, on the other hand, it may lead to keen competitiveness, pugnacity, loneliness and confusion of generations.

With older siblings acting in parental roles, the younger child may form close attachments which are irregularly disrupted by the many changes in the lives of the "auxiliary parents." The elder children in a large family may be mature in the way of taking responsibility and doing chores, but may have missed developing such inner resources as imagination, generosity, and spontaneity.

A small family may instill in the child a strict conscience, and rigid patterns of relating to authority because of the absence of the moderating influence of other siblings. There is also the danger of narrow family alliances; e.g., father-daughter, mother-son, which limit a broader identification with both parents' gender roles and those of siblings.

Special family experiences need to be included in any assessment. The following events—when a child has died, a parent is chronically ill, the family has moved frequently, or the children vacation with certain relatives —differentiate these families from the family unit that has never experienced loss or separation. Obviously the effect of hospitalization on individual families will also differ.

If the professional keeps in mind the average characteristics for a particular patient with respect to culture, economic condition, and family unit characteristics, he will look for confirmation or differentiation from this expectation. For example, a baby who had failed to thrive, required multiple admissions and diagnostic procedures before the staff became aware that his eating and sleeping arrangements in a culture-of-poverty were affecting his growth. When these were altered the child prospered.

There are still such family constellations (occurring in all cultures) as: the emotional, the deceptive, the punitive-depriving, the magical, the culturally poor, the overprotective, the militantly religious and the well-adapted. The following are descriptions of these family types:

Emotional Family

The emotional family is noted by its histrionics and mood swings. In the hospital, family members mill about the corridors and reception areas implying to the child that his condition must be serious. The parents themselves, under pressure by grandparents and relatives, are unable to shield their child from the alarming interactions with the extended family. Because the nuclear family has been splintered, an atmosphere of crisis takes over. Gossip goes on and a worried pall hangs over everyone. Frequently, the occasion is used for mutual closeness and conviviality instead of being used to give support to the child. Bedside and corridor vigils are common, as are efforts to bring in home cooked meals. Food becomes a major symbol for showing love for the child and hostility toward the staff.

The family's efforts to insulate him can only be interpreted by the child as their distrust of the hospital environment. This severely limits the child's adaptation. It takes firmness and patience for the staff to deal with these well-meaning though disrupting people. Reliance on hospital rules helps to set limits. Lengthy explanations of medical procedures or mental health needs of children are of no avail. Visiting hours for the extended family need to be curbed. The parents need much support toward keeping the nuclear family functioning despite the rest of their family. For this end, a good relationship with a staff person is crucial. Often contact with these parents reveals that they both revere and fear one particular family figure who is directing the others. They are usually grateful for any assistance in managing this individual.

Progress with this family is shown by a greater sense of calm, less frenetic handling of the child by relatives, and a diminishing number of visitors.

The Deceptive Family

The deceptive family makes untrue statements to the child regarding his illness. Commonly information about the hospitalization is withheld such as the timing of the trip to the hospital, the length of stay, and what will be done medically. Treatment is usually presented as if it were an amusement park experience. These attitudes affect the child severely. With respect to his family relationships, there may develop feelings of unease, confusion, and betrayal along with loss of the ability to trust any adults. Parents' reactions are complex. They think that concealing facts will diminish the pain for the child. They also seek to spare themselves awareness of the truth. These parents often make impossible promises as to the outcome of treatment while failing to discuss with the child what he expects: To one child hospitalization might mean changing size, or acquiring the ability to hit home runs, or being able to see better. The disappointments subsequent to surgery occur just at the time the child needs security the most—during the painful early convalescence.

These family patterns can be inadvertently supported when the staff purposely avoids intervening, knowing how unpleasant the encounter may be. Emboldened by the staff's silence, the family may try to enlist the staff in tricking the child. At times these families even deceive themselves, and so hide from the truth that they believe their own wishes; e.g., a child in a deep coma will be reported by a parent to be communicating.

In spite of the help these families need, they can be quite provocative and so alienate people around them as to prevent counsel. The staff's awareness of their own reaction may help them to give this family more empathy than anger. The parents may stop deceiving themselves for a while if they discuss the long range results. The children should be talked to diplomatically so that although they learn the truth, they do not become enraged with their families. If the parents' attitude changes, and they want the child to know the facts, they will need assistance. It may be the first time they have admitted fallibility to the child. Another dilemma for the parents to face is how to apologize with dignity, while maintaining the child's confidence. They might be helped to say: "We believed that keeping this from you was in your interest, but now we see that our loving wish to protect you was mistaken. Our intentions though good, only resulted in confusing you and making you doubt our words. We're sorry. There are things you want to ask about. We think we'll be able to answer them." Once parents tell the truth, they need to be shown the happy effects on the child—more openness and more lively interchanges.

The Punitive-Depriving Family

Another family constellation is one that could be called the punitive-depriving one. Threatened or actual physical abuse is a favored method of discipline. Children are made to tow the line and to submit. The mother's fear of spoiling the child is seen by her reluctance to hold and comfort him. The father is either hostile or withdrawn, and often uses alcohol. These children can do nothing right except keep out of the way of grownups. Parents see the staff as indulgent and permissive, and anticipate discipline problems when the child returns home. They are jealous that while in the hospital the child will become attached to a caring person who is kind and generous.

Sickness to these parents implies some new calamity which they meet with anger. This family pattern maintains egocentric thinking beyond the age of 6 years (when it usually ebbs). The child is accustomed to the idea that illness is caused by personal actions and is a punishment for badness. Because he is so overcontrolled and harassed by rules at home, the child becomes confused and filled with anxiety when he goes into the different and less structured situation of the hospital. The child convinced that he is being punished does not understand leniency and expects a surprise attack.

Before a plan is made to help these families, the dynamics of their behavior should be known to the staff. The parents are doing to their children what their parents did to them. The mothers accustomed to hardship are long-suffering and have low self-esteem. They were taught to expect a bleak existence. The fathers were infantilized and overcontrolled by mothers who were angry at men and uncomfortable with the manly assertiveness in their sons. Because they were not cherished and accepted as children, these men and women cannot offer tender forms of love to their offspring.

Suggestions for helping these families while in the hospital setting are the following:

On arrival, these children require clear simple information as to what is expected, and consistent assignment to a staff person who should offer a low-keyed verbal relationship. These children suspect adults who are overly warm. The mother needs to be indulged and respected. She might then allow similar kindness to be offered to her child. The staff needs to ask the mother what she does for pleasure and to encourage her to have a more fulfilled life. This will make her less jealous and less resentful when her child is treated as an individual. Improvement in both mother and child is signalled by increasing expressivity, joking, rebelliousness and candor. The main peril of carrying out the hospital plan is the initial staff hostility, which frequently develops when the rejecting and dehumanizing behavior of these parents is observed. The staff in their efforts to rescue these waif-like children may be rude and judgmental—unnecessarily insulting the parents, who need more pity than punishment.

The Magical-Thinking Family

The family that uses magical-thinking to deal with stress may see sickness as an omen of bad things to come, as a signal of God's displeasure, or fate. Fundamentally suspicious of the majority culture, this family's thinking heightens the child's fear (especially of death) in the hospital and increases his mistrust of outsiders—represented by medical and nursing staff. The child craves emblems and objects to protect him from further damage. Mother's scarf or father's keys can give him much comfort. The infrequency of abstract thinking may be noticed. The child may pray to certain secret protectors for safety. The staff needs to be particularly careful that these families do not hear snippets of frightening medical talk.

Parents in these families are often docile and childlike. They ask for detailed instructions, which are followed reverentially. Whatever is said must be clear. These parents do best when they can call on the doctor to answer questions. Conditional statements such as—if fever goes up two degrees give more aspirin—only tend to confuse the parents. The staff needs to be vigilant since a too literal interpretation of directions may be counterproductive. Also when speaking with the child, simple direct language, avoiding complex abstractions, is best. One or two professionals should communicate all information to the family, as even slight vocabulary differences will seem to represent hidden dangers against which they have to guard.

The staff should be pleased when they hear that they are included in daily prayers. This shows that the staff is thought of as friends; on the other hand, this may indicate the family believes the staff needs "outside" help.

The Culture-of-Poverty Family

The culture-of-poverty family is characterized by a fatalistic, present-oriented, authoritarian outlook. Male and female roles are rigidly defined. One finds a distrust of outsiders, whose behavior is considered unpredictable and is judged on its immediate impact. Low self-esteem leads these families to have little belief in their own coping capacities.[5] Generally, there is limited verbal communication, passive attitudes toward mastering new experiences, and ignorance of body physiology. The mother is chief caretaker with the father often absent. When present he can be harsh in his interactions within the family. Both parents have volatile tempers.

High marital conflict and frequent family breakdown are present along with a low educational level and alienation among family members. There is a defeatist attitude toward the future. Generally, families of a lower social class are oriented to child rearing by overpowering the small person who can submit, rebel or withdraw. Without clear-cut authority, these people become anxious and defensively hostile. (See chart, page 44.) They are not accustomed to a democratic, inclusive form of treatment.

Children in this environment behave impulsively without regard for the deeper responsibility of their actions. They often project blame to others rather than seeing what role they play in the situation; thus a main objective for them is to keep from getting caught. When the children annoy their parents they suffer ridicule and capriciously harsh discipline. The parents rely on physical rather than verbal control of behavior, and encourage and discourage alternatively, assertiveness in their children. Because of previous disappointments and identification with role models who avoid the unexpected, these children are reluctant to encounter new experiences. Instead they become anxious and aggressive when confronted by the novel. In fact, the continuous exposure to violent changes in atmosphere prevents an adaptive tolerance for anxiety. Turbulence can be integrated only in small doses. Consequently, these children panic easily as shown by their hyperactivity.

The staff needs to understand that their middle class values are inappropriate in the management of these families. Wherever hospital personnel are verbal, future-oriented, and permissive, these children will rapidly become unruly and disruptive. Conversely, to use an authoritarian power-oriented approach only perpetuates their maladaptive style.

The professional who at the outset is able to be sensibly authoritarian is usually the one best able to instruct these families as well as best able to allay their fears. Lengthy discussions, talk of possible eventualities, and discussion of the genetic implications of illness are not relevant. The earliest sign of change in these families may be their increasing verbalization, and lessening of pessimism about the future. Early improvement in the child is shown by more purposeful behavior; i.e., greater attention span and frustration tolerance.

In time the parents' domination of the children lessens. This lessening of domination can be instigated by the staff in various ways so that the child is seen as an individual whose behavior is motivated by multiple factors. Parents can observe how staff interact with children and can be told about the child's unique and praiseworthy characteristics. They can learn other methods of discipline,[6] the best being to give praise for what is desired behavior and to disregard what is undesirable. The next best method of discipline is through the child's identification with parental attitudes and actions.

The Overprotective Family

The ambitious, overprotective family indulges the child and makes him feel entitled to the gratification of every whim.[7] The parents, often self-

CHILD-REARING AND FAMILY LIFE PATTERNS REPORTED TO BE MORE CHARACTERISTIC OF FAMILIES OF CHILDREN WHO ARE EMOTIONALLY HEALTHY COMPARED WITH RELEVANT PATTERNS REPORTED TO BE MORE CHARACTERISTIC OF VERY POOR FAMILIES*

EMOTIONALLY HEALTHY CHILDREN

1. Respect for child as individual whose behavior is caused by a multiple of factors. Acceptance of own role in events that occur.

2. Commitment to slow development of child from infancy to maturity; stresses and pressures of each stage accepted by parent because of perceived worth of ultimate goal of raising "happy," successful son or daughter.

3. Relative sense of competence in handling child's behavior.

4. Discipline chiefly verbal, mild, reasonable, consistent, based on needs of child and family and of society; more emphasis on rewarding good behavior than on punishing bad behavior.

5. Open, free, verbal communication between parent and child; control largely verbal.

6. Democratic rather than autocratic or laissez-faire methods of rearing, with both parents in equalitarian but not necessarily interchangeable roles. Companionship between parents and children.

POVERTY LIFE STYLES

1. Misbehavior regarded as such in terms of concrete pragmatic outcomes; reasons for behavior not considered. Projection of blame on others.

2. Lack of goal commitment and of belief in long-range success; a main object for parent and child is to "keep out of trouble"; orientation toward fatalism, impulse gratification, and sense of alienation.

3. Sense of powerlessness in handling children's behavior, as well as in other areas.

4. Discipline harsh, inconsistent, physical, makes use of ridicule; punishment based on whether child's behavior does or does not annoy parent.

5. Limited verbal communication; control largely physical.

6. Authoritarian rearing methods; mother chief child-care agent; father, when in home, mainly punitive figure. Little support and acceptance of child as an individual.

7. Parents view selves as generally competent adults and are generally satisfied with themselves and their situation.

8. Intimate, expressive, warm relationship between parent and child, allowing for gradually increasing independence. Sense of continuing parental responsibility.

9. Free verbal communication about sex, acceptance of child's sex needs, channeling of sex drive through "healthy" psychological defenses, acceptance of slow growth toward impulse control and sex satisfaction in marriage; sex education by both father and mother.

10. Acceptance of child's drive for aggression but channeling it into socially approved outlets.

11. In favor of new experiences; flexible.

12. Happiness of parental marriage.

7. Low parental self-esteem, sense of defeat.

8. Large families; more impulsive, narcissistic parent behavior. Orientation to "excitement." Abrupt, early yielding of independence.

9. Repressive, punitive attitude about sex, sex questioning, and experimentation. Sex viewed as exploitative relationship.

10. Alternating encouragement and restriction of aggression, primarily related to consequences of aggression for parents.

11. Distrust of new experiences. Constricted life, rigidity.

12. High rates of marital conflict and family breakdown.

* Chilman, C. S.: Growing Up Poor. Washington, D.C., U.S. Department of Health, Education, and Welfare, 1966.

sacrificing, live for the future when the child will bring credit to them. The child as the standard-bearer of the family, embodies all their hopes for a better, more perfect image of themselves. Though this family appears to be child-centered as the child is "given everything," it really is achievement oriented. In the hospital, the parents show a confusion of their own needs and those of the child by wanting a quick cure so the child can resume the "horse race" of life. This attitude leads them to frequent checking on the staff to assure themselves that their future investment is safe. There is latent hostility toward the child for being ill and interfering with their plans for his attainments.

The best management of this family is to begin by impressing them with staff competence, and letting them know everyone is equally anxious and desirous of a quick cure. Praise should be given for how well the family has coped with the illness. Then limits need to be set for the parents and their frequently overindulged children. Their anxiety will not abate until they understand the necessity of hospital regulations and realize the trustworthiness of the staff.

Careful explanations about diagnostic and therapeutic procedures are helpful, provided parents listen and do not use the knowledge to compete with professionals in the treatment of their child. Compliments for the staff signal a change in attitude and a lower anxiety. However, the staff must be cautious and not accept compliments; instead they should turn them around and tell the parents, "You're so gracious but really, you've had the hardest part of the job—longest and most taxing." To accept a compliment without returning the courtesy can mislead, because parents may have mixed motives.

Children from these families are often openly aggressive and demanding, and see themselves as the equals of adults. The parents' behavior toward the staff only reinforces the child's negative, petulant, testy attitudes. Eventually there is a confrontation in which someone from the staff tells the child that in the hospital he must live by the regulations, though once at home, he can return to his usual bossiness. Amazingly, this is usually sufficient to curb the more obnoxious actions. If the child persists in his selfishness, variations of the GOLDEN RULE can be tried—"If you treat people this way they will do the same to you"; or, "How can you expect consideration and warmth when you don't give them?" In addition, when these children show the least change toward being more pleasant, this improvement should be quickly, though casually acknowledged.

The Family Whose Religion Interferes With Treatment

The family whose religious principles conflict with medical authority creates special difficulties for their hospitalized children. If they were to agree to medical or surgical treatment, their beliefs would be violated. Special difficulties are mistrust, fear, and withdrawal in the child, along with clinging to the parents. The staff should try to persuade them of the child's best medical interests, though the parents' right to their own beliefs must be respected. When parents become vehement in their rejection of applied science, this may cause staff resentment which further augments the child's anxiety.

Where there is close rapport with parents and respect for their beliefs, the child may begin to trust the staff. The child needs much support to develop a sense of security in the hospital. In chronic illness, parents should be informed of the expectation for future hospitalizations so that whatever consent they give for treatment can be applied subsequently. This obviates the necessity of repetitive discussion. When parents continue to refuse medical intervention, a medical-legal expert is helpful to determine the child's rights to adequate treatment. Court action may be involved, because these parents cannot compromise their beliefs, but will surrender to overwhelming secular authority. Outside resources should be used, such as the clergy of their denomination. Every attempt should be made to avoid recourse to litigation.

The Best Adapted Family[8,9]

The best adapted family is one that uses mild, firm, consistent discipline, is rational, evidence-oriented, and objective. It looks to the future goals, is self-confident, trustful and enjoys new experience. Democratic and equalitarian, this family uses extensive verbal communication—valuing complexity and abstractions. Human behavior is seen as developmental in nature and having many causes. There is high self-esteem, a belief in one's own coping capacity, and an active attitude. Each child is seen as separate and unique and is given consistent support and gradual training for independence.

The marriage is harmonious with both parents having achieved occupational and educational success. There is an intimate, expressive, warm relationship between parent and child; sexual and aggressive drives are accepted and channeled toward approved outlets and impulse control.

The hospitalized child from this family will not be immune to fears or regressive behaviors, but after the age of four will be able to adapt to stresses provided there are adequate mother substitutes and a secure, warm environment.

These children are inquisitive and imaginative. Conversations adequate for their age, play, and instruction will fortify them for what is to be done to their bodies. The hospitalization becomes a challenge to be met and conquered—thus adding to their sense of competence and confidence.

What often distinguishes these families is their ability to preserve the usual relationship despite the separation and anxiety due to illness. In fact the relationship may gain added depth for their having experienced together a serious health crisis.

THE FAMILY DIAGNOSTIC INTERVIEW

Although family diagnosis is usually the prerogative of the psychiatrist and social worker, other pediatric professionals who move to areas where these resource people are not available may find techniques of family diagnostic interview worthwhile.[10] Indeed, when extensive facilities are lacking or special consultants unavailable, anyone working with children will find this skill a necessity.

Much of the original work for family diagnosis was done with very disturbed patients and their families. Findings indicated severe disturbances in communication—the double bind and pseudo-mutual modes of interaction leading to perplexity.* These were found particularly in families having a schizophrenic patient. However, these pathologic patterns can exist to a lesser degree in any family. Abnormal communication may exist in any of the previously mentioned family types.

To conduct a productive family diagnosis, all members of the family group need to be present. This would include nonrelatives if they play a significant role, or exclude close relations if they are uninvolved.

---

* Pseudo-mutuality is the type of communication in a family where expression of conflict is not permitted and children are not differentiated from the parents and each other.

Double bind is a type of communication from an important person in the form of two messages, one denying the other. The child is forced to respond to a contradiction or incongruity.

Perplexity is the mental state resulting from being placed in pseudo-mutual or double bind situations.

If the family as a group is facing some task that requires coping (i.e., deprivation and loss, birth or addition of a new member, illness, and loss of physical powers), this would emerge during a conference. Then certain commonly found family interactional patterns should be noted such as:

the family that expresses intimacy through fighting. One family regularly created scenes in the public areas of the hospital while waiting emergency treatment for their asthmatic son.

the family that utilizes the occasion of a neutral leader to say things that they are too frightened to say to each other.

the family that scapegoats; e.g., one person is assigned a "sick" role.

the family that uses family myths; e.g., one family believed that the father was a tyrant until they saw that he was merely carrying out the orders of the grandmother.

the family that expects individual needs to be gratified without those needs being openly stated.

the family that uses "push-pull" patterns—where one member regularly provokes another to having a certain reaction.

Findings from family conferences reflect their uniqueness. From the diagnostic interview the family interactional pattern becomes clear. This added to the type of family (described above as emotional, magical, etc.) the size of family and its development as a unit, will encompass the major part of a child's world. In general, for professionals there is a shift from seeing only the patient to seeing the latter in his usual habitat. One look at the way a child is treated by different family members is worth hours of close interview of individuals. Since doctors and nurses may have a predilection to treat the patient in vacuo and to leave the family to the social worker, they need to experience interaction with this social unit in their preparation for working in a community setting. Social workers may not always be available; thus it is necessary for medically trained people to have experience in these areas.

Finally, the development of professional staff occurs where intimate contact with other ways of living has a vividness and impact. Intensive academic training may alienate the student and recent graduate from his and her own family and certainly from families of different origins. In becoming professional there is a removal from a family setting not only because of student life, but also because the student frequently surpasses his family's educational achievement. This can lead the professional to be hypercritical of the family as an organization.

REFERENCES

1. Spiegel, J. P.: Cultural strain, family role patterns, and intrapsychic conflict. *In* Howells, J. G.: Theory and Practice of Family Psychiatry. New York, Brunner/Mazel, 1971.

2. Erikson, E. H.: Childhood and Society. ed. 2, pp. 277-325. New York, W. W. Norton, 1963.

3. Report of the Joint Commission on Mental Health of Children: Crisis in Child Mental Health. pp. 264-265. New York, Harper & Row, 1969.

4. Hollingshead, A., and Redlich, F.: Social Class and Mental Illness. Chapters 4 and 7, New York, John Wiley & Sons, 1958.

5. Reissman, F.: The Culturally Deprived Child. pp. 36-48. New York, Harper & Row, 1962.

6. Becker, W. C.: Consequences of different kinds of parental discipline. *In* Hoffman, M. L., and Hoffman, L. W. (eds.): Review of Child Development Research, vol. 1. New York, Russell Sage Foundation, 1964.

7. Levy, D. M.: Maternal Overprotection. pp. 161-199. New York, W. W. Norton, 1966.

8. Ackerman, N. W.: The Psychodynamics of Family Life: Diagnosis and Treatment of Family Relationships. pp. 3-25. New York, Basic Books, 1958.

9. Lidz, T.: The Family and Human Adaptation. pp. 39-113. New York, International Universities Press, 1963.

10. Caplan, G.: An approach to the study of family mental health. *In* Galdston, I. (ed.): The Family, A Focal Point in Health Education. New York, International Universities Press, 1961.

BIBLIOGRAPHY

Ackerman, N. W.: Treating the Troubled Family. New York, Basic Books, 1966.

Clausen, J. A.: Family structure, socialization and personality. *In* Hoffman, L. W., and Hoffman, M. L. (eds.): Review of Child Development Research. vol. 2. New York, Russell Sage Foundation, 1966.

Goldfarb, W., *et al.:* The concept of maternal perplexity. *In* Anthony, E. J., and Benedek, T. (eds.): Parenthood, Its Psychology and Psycopathology. Boston, Little, Brown & Co., 1970.

Greenblatt M., *et al.:* Poverty and mental health: implications for training. Psychiat. Res. Rep. Amer. Psychiat. Ass., *21*:151, 1967.

Harrison, S. I., *et al.:* Social class and mental illness in children: choice of treatment. Arch. Gen. Psychiat., *13*:411, 1965.

Irelan, L. (ed.): Low-income Life Styles. Washington, D.C., Dept of Health, Education and Welfare, 1966.

Lidz, T., *et al.:* Schism and skew in the families of schizophrenics. *In* Bell, N. W., and Vogel, E. F. (eds.): Modern Introduction To The Family. rev. ed. New York, The Free Press, 1968.

Lolli, G., *et al.:* Alcohol in Italian Culture. New Haven, Conn., College and University Press, 1958.

McDermott, J. F., *et al.:* Social class and mental illness in children. The diagnosis of organicity and mental retardation. J. Amer. Acad. Child Psychiat., *6*:309, 1967.

McDonald, N. F., and Adams, P. L.: The psychotherapeutic workability of the poor. J. Amer. Acad. Child Psychiat., *6*:663, 1967.

Report of the Joint Commission on Mental Health of Children: Crisis in Child Mental Health: Challenge for the 1970's. Chap. 2. Contemporary American society: its impact on the mental health of children and youth. Chap. 4. Poverty and mental health. New York, Harper & Row, 1969.

Snyder, C. R.: Alcohol and the Jews. New Haven, Conn., College and University Press, 1958.

Szurek, S., Johnson, A., and Falstein, E.: Collaborative psychiatric treatment of parent-child problems. Amer. J. Orthopsychiat., *12*:511, 1942.

Watzlawick, P.: A review of the double bind theory. *In* Howells, J. G. (ed.):

Theory and Practice of Family Psychiatry. New York, Brunner/Mazel, 1971.

Weakland, J. H.: The "double-bind" hypothesis of schizophrenia and three-party interaction. *In* Jackson, D. D. (ed.): The Etiology of Schizophrenia. New York, Basic Books, 1960.

Wynne, L. C., *et al.:* Pseudo-mutuality in the family relations of schizophrenics. *In* Bell, N. W., and Vogel, E. F. (eds.): Modern Introduction To The Family. rev. ed. New York, The Free Press, 1960.

4

Child, Parent, Staff Interactions

THE INTERVIEW

The ability to conduct a competent interview is a basic skill useful in any area of professional life. The objective is to derive relevant and reliable information in a manner both efficient and considerate. To do this, one needs a planned approach along with a sensitive ear in order to survey the broad areas of the patient's life without missing the subtleties. Obviously, an effective grasp of a patient's life situation can directly affect the quality of his management. Feeling tones, incidental remarks, and body language can give clues to the most meaningful attitudes and experiences. The following diagnostic procedure should not be confused with the more typical medical history taking which all too often approximates an interrogation for purposes of filling in a checklist. Such an inventory dehumanizes the process. The attempt here is to revise this traditional model.

The first step for an interviewer to keep in mind when seeing a child and his family is that this may not be the family's initial experience with a caretaker or professional. It is essential for the interviewer to discover the family's past relationships with medical personnel and the impressions they made. Although the chief complaint and present problem are important medically, knowing the child's previous encounters would justify the extra effort to obtain this information because undoubtedly, the present reaction is strongly colored by earlier contacts.

> Richard, an obese teenager hitherto known by the staff as "the slob," had a previous colectomy during which his appendix was removed as a part of the standard operating procedure; however, they removed it without his knowledge. Now he was resisting further surgery—revision of the colectomy and an ileostomy. He was also ready to sign out of the hospital. His submissive parents were powerless to influence him. He was belligerently and stubbornly silent with the pediatrician; however, he gave clues to several staff members which indicated his deep sense of having

been betrayed, and his mistrust of surgery (for what might be done to him without his permission). Fortunately, one of the members of the original surgical group responsible for the removal of his appendix was invited to attend an emergency meeting of the mental health team. This doctor then reviewed with Richard the previous surgery, and tendered an apology for the oversight of not informing him of the appendectomy. They also discussed in detail the impending surgery. Richard was proud of his assertiveness and pleased with his importance; therefore, the outcome of this rapport and belated apology led to his consenting to surgery.

Mrs. D. previously had multiple hospitalizations and openly complained to the nurses about past mistakes doctors had made in her care. Yet she was bewildered by her son's excessive fears about hospitalization and his aversion to doctors and nurses because he had never been in a hospital. Discovery of his mother's influence regarding medical "mistreatment" allowed the staff to intervene successfully. At first he was encouraged to describe his knowledge of hospitals; then to describe what would happen as he imagined it. Finally, his actual illness was described to him, and it was emphasized that he had a different diagnosis than his mother. He learned also that his treatment and recovery would not be the same as hers.

The interviewer should avoid making promises that cannot be fulfilled or making predictions that cannot be anticipated with certainty. Experiences over the years have shown the need for caution in giving to the child ideas that lead to magical expectation of improvement or cure. Parents out of guilt and doctors out of anxiety, despite the best of intentions, can (particularly with preschoolers) have the child imagining strange consequences—to become muscular and stronger than a sibling, to be more acceptable to parents, to be taller. Unreal hopes are also likely to occur in the child who is confused on arrival at the hospital because of inadequate preparation.

Nonetheless, even with the parent's observance of this caution, a child often develops his own notions of what will happen to him after hospitalization. These need to become known to the staff. Children will have fantasies particular to their age. (See *Preoperative fantasies*, pages 73–75.)

Deaths in the family that were preceded by hospitalization, can be associated in the child's mind in such a way as to cause panic at the prospect of a severe illness. In this case it is because the child (under 6) may associate going to the hospital with a morbid outcome, particularly—mutilation.

The above possibilites need to be considered before a formal interview takes place. In this first phase, the all important rapport with the child and family needs to be solidified before any further information is solicited. Naturally, the physician and nurse in charge must identify themselves and explain the roles of subordinate and paraprofessionals.

The next step for the interviewer is to decide on the general areas to be covered by the interview—these differ with various syndromes. For example, in the immediate posttrauma period for a burned child, interest in the safety of the home, the guilt of parents, and the circumstances of the accident, would be more pertinent to elucidate than whether the child has a history of the common childhood illnesses, or whether he is usually battling with a certain sibling. With the readmission of an asthmatic, the interviewer should be alert for triggering events such as arguments, new people in the home, separations, and recent lapses in the home treatment of minor respiratory ailments.

After considering the broad areas to be covered, parents should be asked such open-ended questions as: "How have things been with your family these last few weeks? What has gone on? How did this happen? When did you first notice a change in the child's health and what happened after that? What should we know that would help us make your child more comfortable in the hospital? Who and what will he miss by being away from home? What are his likeable qualities?"

People prefer to say things in their own way. These opening questions make that possible. As long as the answers they give appear to have relevance to the management of the child, parents welcome the opportunity to be candid about their lives.

The third step for the interviewer is to take the usual, careful medical interview which contains details on present illness, history, review of systems, physical examination, and diagnosis.

The fourth step should be taken by that interviewer who has the beginnings of a solid relationship with the family and intends to continue developing it. For this step he follows up leads from the preceding steps and begins to inquire about issues that may be threatening. Such things asked about are omissions, overt and covert complaints, topics glossed over, and any oddities. For example, the response may be significant— if the only thing Johnny is missing is the vacuum cleaner, if the father is not mentioned, if it is passingly stated that things have been awful for months, or if the obvious hardships of a chronic illness are denied.

Fifth, it is highly desirable to interview others in the same family by using this general approach. The assessments described in Chapter 3 are brought in at this time. (See The Family Diagnostic Interview, page 48.)

Sixth, the interviewer should explore specific issues generally known to challenge and upset most individuals and families. These issues often form the foci of further difficulties. Examples of nonthreatening inquiries which elicit information and uncover problem areas are: "Who is supportive in the environment? To whom do you turn when you need help? Who helps with the children? How do the different individuals in the family respond to the illness? Does the family as a group find stressful events pulling them together or apart? Are there typical difficulties? Is this child different from siblings or cousins? What has been his most difficult area of growing up? How do you think this illness came about? What do other members of the family think about how the illness started? Does this illness bring relatives into the family who are not usually seen? Do you like this? How are the remaining children being cared for? What do they know of the patient's illness and about hospitals? Is this illness interfering with plans the family has made (economically, geographically and socially)?"

Also much valuable information for the effective management of the child can be learned by the following interview questions: "Is the marriage harmonious? What is the prevailing form of punishment? Do the parents have a life of their own? What is the overall emotional atmosphere? How secure is the family financially? What are their pastimes? Was the patient born at a convenient time in the family history?"

The above questions elicit information that leads to the formation of a judgment about the family adaptation in the past and in the present. Furthermore, with some degree of confidence, the family's capacity to take in new information and follow through on instructions can be predicted. Prior to discharge, plans could thus be made regarding the type of help specific to carrying out a therapeutic regimen—visiting nurse, homemaker, social worker and outpatient care. These seven steps give the initial guidelines and direction to the mental health team and to everyone in the pediatric unit who interacts with this patient and his family during their first days in the hospital. This interview procedure should be applied with each readmission as new family experiences may have caused significant changes in the child's needs.

ENCOUNTERS OF STAFF WITH PARENTS WHO "ROOM-IN" AND PARTICIPATE IN CHILD CARE

Upon a child's admission to the hospital, one of the great concerns of parents—visiting and rooming-in privileges—has been arbitrarily settled according to the policies of the institution. Despite research findings that indicate conclusively the damaging effects on young children of separation from their mothers,[1,2,3] the application of this knowledge is lacking in most pediatric departments, and the merits of parent participation in the care of hospitalized children remains a controversial issue.

However, there is an increasing tendency in many communities to challenge the archaic regulations that prevent close interaction of families during periods of stress. Existing knowledge favors more flexible approaches. Also for a growing number of pediatric personnel, the issue is no longer whether it is wise to permit extensive interaction of families during hospitalization, but rather, how this interaction can be accomplished in the light of inadequate facilities.

Drawbacks to this trend are noteworthy. Few institutions today are sufficiently modern and spacious to accommodate comfortably the presence of family members and their personal effects. The staff frequently complains that it takes time and effort to answer questions, to teach child care, and to tolerate the supervising and challenging statements of parents.

Fortunately the disadvantages of time, space, and staff-family conflict are balanced by the obvious positive aspects. Evidence of these positive aspects is given by the absence of separation anxiety as described by Robertson*; the greater sense of security children feel when accompanied by their parents; the comfort mothers give to one another and the greater absorption of the teaching program by these families. Also persuasive of this philosophy is the opportunity it affords for evaluation of the mother-child and other family relationships.

> Davey, 9 months old, was admitted to the hospital because he was failing to thrive. During the admission interview, the pediatrician observed a loving, concerned mother who derived gratification from caring for her son. Her only complaint was the amount of time each meal required. Subsequent observations of the mother as she participated in his care during the following week, altered

* See Phases of Separation Anxiety, page 66.

the initial impression. The feeding process as described by the staff consisted of a 1½ hour "shooting-in" process; that is, the mother took aim from a distance of a few inches and threw food at the infant's mouth. Very little food hit the target. Repeatedly the mother berated the nurses for the ease in which they fed the child successfully, although they made every effort to underplay their success (in order to minimize the mother's jealousy). Their suggestions only frustrated this mother and confirmed her inadequacy to herself and to others. On two occasions Mrs. M. revealed her deeper concerns—disappointment over the sex of the child and his resemblance to his father. These findings altered the approach in this case. Instead of proceeding with medical investigation of each physiologic system, as was planned for Davey, the staff realized the mother needed assistance to resolve her fear and dislike of males and to develop confidence in the maternal role. She was encouraged to see a social worker regularly.

When a parent program is to be established, thoughts on the prerequisites can avoid unnecessary resistance later on. A pilot effort in a small pediatric unit is one way to find out the impediments to this idea. Before hospitalization or during the admission interview, parents can be informed of an existing program for young children (typically under 6, although age should not be a barrier when children are critically ill). The types of activities in which the staff would welcome family involvement with patients need to be made clear; e.g., bathing, dressing, feeding, accompanying to diagnostic procedures, participating in recreation, preparing for bed, and assisting with procedures which will eventually require home follow-up.

Caution should be taken to avoid arousal of guilt in a mother who already has conflicts about separating from her child because of responsibilities to her other siblings. Also to be avoided is the participation of parents whose prolonged presence in the hospital life stifles the patient's involvement with peers, and interferes generally with his adjustment.

Henrietta, age 14, balked at her parent's continuous presence during the day and her mother's sleeping in her room overnight. She was delighted when the staff intervened on her behalf by convincing her family of her good adjustment in the hospital. With this assurance they were able to leave this budding adolescent to her own resources, for long periods.

Harry, age 7, was bewildered by his mother's concentrated attention. Normally, he was cared for by servants and saw his parents at rigidly scheduled periods during the day. After his admission, his mother was convinced by other parents of the importance of her participation. She complied with obvious discomfort. This unfortunately worked against Harry, who believed that he must be sicker than he thought to warrant such unfamiliar togetherness. Discussion with Mrs. B. regarding the advisability of a regular visiting pattern for children in Harry's age group, brought immediate relief for this mother who was released from an imposed maternal role; consequently, her absence allowed him to seek out friends, and a mother substitute from the nursing staff.

While the majority of parents pose little difficulty for the staff, the few who become nuisances are easily remembered and supply the evidence for personnel who oppose the increased parent participation. The potential for staff-family conflict is great—considering the pressures under which medical staffs work, and the anxieties of parents with sick children. Not to be forgotten is the fact that many individuals are difficult even under ideal situations. In stress everyone demonstrates an intensified version of his everyday self; consequently illness shows us people at their best or at their worst. Realistically then, staff and parents need to be protected by enlightened policies and guidelines that are designed to curb interpersonal friction, and permit parent programs and the usual routines of ward management to continue.

Firsthand experience with parents who participate in child care or stay overnight is persuasive of the importance of having the policies and limits of family involvement clearly specified in writing. A brochure prepared for parents stating what to expect, often prevents major collisions with staff. The pediatric department needs to support the philosophy that overnight accommodations are made available because the staff recognizes that hospitalization is less traumatic for young children when a family member is consistently present, and this conviction has prompted the institution to initiate a parent program in the face of inadequate structural facilities. A realistic description of accommodations—sleeping, bathing, and dining arrangements—is essential. Departments can rarely offer the conveniences of home. An honest presentation would influence parent's expectations and curtail the number of complaints regarding the facilities. At the outset, those individuals who require the kind of services that are beyond the staff's capacity, could be smoothly discouraged from rooming-in.

Parents need to know that regardless of their presence or absence, medical and nursing personnel observe their child and carry out procedures on a 24-hour basis; that whenever indicated they will enter the child's room, possibly disturbing a parent sleeping in the same room. It must be understood that the staff assumes responsibility for the child's welfare even though some procedures are delegated to the parents.

A guide to parents needs to include the regulations which make for harmonious living conditions with children, other parents, and staff. These regulations are often neglected until they become a problem— proper attire (nudity in public areas causes embarrassment for everyone), smoking and alcoholic restrictions, and the number of family members or guests allowed for one patient. When limits are set early, there is less likelihood for rules to be abused.

Rules, of course, are designed to facilitate the smooth functioning of a program; yet they must be flexibly applied. It may be just as appropriate to withdraw privileges as it may be to increase them in the interests of patient care.

> The evening nurse on a busy private unit found herself the scapegoat for a number of anxious mothers after a seemingly minor incident. This occurred when Mrs. Z. returned from dinner to find her infant's diapers soiled. She immediately sought out the nurse in charge and berated her for her negligence. The nurse replied, not too pleasantly, that mothers were permitted to room-in with the understanding that they participate in their child's care; that other more urgent matters required her attention; and that she expected Mrs. Z. to cooperate. However, cooperation was not this mother's game—retaliation was. The tale of the nurse's rudeness and incompetence spread rapidly to several mothers whose children were critically ill. They, along with Mrs. Z., decided that they could not safely leave the unit unless one of them remained on guard. The task of the mother in charge was to supervise the nurse and to report her findings to the others regularly by telephone. Before long, no medication or treatment could be delivered without a challenge. A matter of personality conflict between mothers and nurse, now became a situation where patient care was in jeopardy. The mothers' hysteria grew to the point where they were demanding replacement of the nurse.
> Fortunately in this instance, the nurse was particularly competent. It was clear that she had to be supported and that the floor personnel needed to regain the good will and cooperation of Mrs. Z. After many efforts at trying to regain her cooperation by long talks and explanation, to no avail, it was necessary for the head nurse and chief pediatric resident to place firm limits on Mrs. Z. by allowing her to choose between staying in her room or

leaving the hospital altogether. This had a calming effect on Mrs. Z. The other mothers required an intense group session with the staff before they were convinced that their children were well cared for. Mrs. Z., a few days later, appealed to her private pediatrician for support. However, as a result of being present at a mental health team conference, he concurred with the staff; thus assuring Mrs. Z. that everyone agreed about her child's requirements, and the excellent quality of nursing care.

In the incident described above, there was no conflict between the staff and the attending pediatrician in resolving the problem, but this is not typical. To avoid unseemly professional conflict, there needs to be a departmental policy, established in advance, that specifies how staff-staff and staff-family conflicts are to be handled. It seems reasonable that the authority should rest with those who bear the brunt of the problem— namely the nursing and medical personnel who manage the unit. Decisions cannot be left to those who disregard the implications for total patient care or ignore the effect the decision has on the direct caretakers of the patient.

Negative aspects of a parent participation program are presented to alert staff to the areas that require advance thought and planning. Success does not depend on the parents' awareness of staff goodwill alone. Goodwill is quickly eroded when, for example, the staff regards parent assistance as a time saver and a way of relieving them of those routine activities that demand little training. They can then expect mothers to complain of being exploited or to believe that their children will not be cared for during their absence because the staff has not approached the patients in the parents' presence. Good feelings are also quickly dissipated when a parent has the attitude that the cost of hospitalization entitles her to personal services beyond medical and nursing care for her child.

Any of these complaints should signal to the staff a need for discussion and reorientation of themselves, the parents, or both.

> A nurse who emerges from the patient's room quite irritated, reports that it takes her longer to instruct a mother in the technique of applying leg bags to urinary drainage tubes than it does to just apply them herself.

> A physical therapist excuses herself for not looking in on a parent and child because she "knows" the mother will call if assistance is needed for the child's exercises. The therapist does not understand that her failure to look in is interpreted as neglect by families; whereas short, conveniently planned appearances

would eventually save her from being interrupted by complaints at inopportune moments.

The staff may come to realize that dissatisfaction of parents usually indicates that they may be asking to be appreciated for their efforts or conveying the need for more support in order to cope with illness and hospitalization. When viewed from this perspective, parent participation can seldom be considered a method of relieving staff shortages. Quite the opposite, parent participation may require more staff, but be well worth it.

While an initial enthusiasm of the staff is sufficient to begin parent participation, enthusiasm is not enough to sustain such a program. Mental health workers (psychiatrist, mental health nurse, social worker or psychologist) need to be available in the treatment team to facilitate communication and mitigate the negative feelings of the staff. Overt and covert attitudes about children and their families should be exposed. It is through multidisciplinary conferences that a sensitive communication system can be maintained. Often, nurses will acknowledge and seek help for their apprehension, angry feelings and sense of depletion in their relationships with patients. Physicians who may spend considerably less time with the children, are correspondingly less involved, though their decisions can have momentous effects. Lacking the satisfactions to be enjoyed from intensively developed interactions with young people, they may not be stimulated toward gaining knowledge of the child's world. Through group discussion a more complete picture of staff-patient-family interaction can be elicited and a unified approach to patient management originated.

> The nurse assigned to Mr. S.'s 10-month-old daughter (who was admitted for treatment of respiratory distress) reported that she found it difficult to understand what was going on with the child's father. He called her to the infant's bedside 4 times within an hour indicating quite innocently that the intravenous infusion had almost stopped. On the last occasion, it occurred to Miss M. that something was amiss when she found that the I.V. clamp was adjusted to obstruct the flow of solution altogether. She asked Mr. S. if anyone else had been in to regulate the infusion. He denied this vehemently. However, another nurse, had seen Mr. S. tampering with the clamp and had stopped him. As the discussion proceeded, other staff members gave more evidence of Mr. S.'s interference in his child's treatment. The previous day Mr. S. was seen removing the restraints from the infant's wrists. When reproached for this action, he became quite defensive—stating

that he would not allow his baby to be tortured in this manner. The nurse asked him if he really understood that the purpose was to keep the baby from pulling the needle out of the vein. He answered by telling her at length about the movie *Spartacus* which he had just viewed, and how he associated the torture scenes with the methods of treatment being given to his daughter by the staff. This discussion temporarily helped him to gain perspective.

Nevertheless the pediatric resident's experience with this family indicated that the difficulty was far from resolved. Shortly before the conference the baby developed an asthmatic attack. An injection of adrenalin was ordered. When a nurse attempted to administer the medication, Mr. S. flung himself across the crib and declared that he would not allow this kind of treatment. While the mother stood by wringing her hands, the father continued with his loud protests. The pediatric resident tried to reason with him and when he failed to convince this man of the necessity for medication, he gave up. He told Mr. S. that he had to take the responsibility for whatever happened. Fortunately for the baby, the attack subsided. Unfortunately for the father, the incident reinforced his distrust of the staff, and as a result his anxiety and bellicosity markedly increased.

Information supplied by the head nurse gave the staff some insight into this man's adaptation in his own life. Because he was a successful business executive, Mr. S. was used to making decisions, issuing orders, and demanding immediate action—in short, always exercising complete control of a situation. His wife remarked that few people ever challenged him. He assumed a similar role in the hospital environment, but now he was a hazard to his child's health.

The staff was unanimous in supporting the following plan: That the head nurse and attending physician on separate occasions (a) acknowledge the father's executive talents and ability to get action in his work situation; (b) sympathize with his need to help his child and with his feelings of helplessness in the hospital; (c) determine father's medical background (if any) and experiences with illness and physicians in the past; (d) elicit father's opinions on the management of child and inquire on what basis he makes the judgment; (e) make it clear that his good intentions are interfering with the child's treatment, and that his behavior indicates he has lost perspective between his own sense of helplessness and that of his child; (f) explain that the medical staff is competent in areas in which he is not and that the staff will be in charge, taking complete responsibility for the medical care— otherwise medical care might not be continued. Not surprisingly, once Mr. S. realized the firm determination, the unity of the staff, and his own overprotection, he acquiesced. Secure in the fact that someone was in charge, he no longer felt that he had to manage the case.

There is another facet of parent participation in patient care which deserves attention. It concerns fundamental interdisciplinary problems which are often aggravated by the presence of persons outside the system. The manner in which nurses and physicians react to complaints made by parents exposes these difficulties. Traditionally, nurses tend to defend the physician's actions and to enhance his reputation in the eyes of the patient and his family. This characteristic behavior is the result of the indoctrination of basic nursing education—supposedly in the interest of the patient. The reverse is not true. Parents' complaints to doctors regarding the work of nurses and other paramedical personnel very often receive support (the excuse being that the customer is always right). Both attitudes of the nurses and doctors are detrimental in managing problems that involve parents as illustrated by the following incident.

> Mrs. B's distrust of the nursing staff became quite apparent when Judd was transferred from the Intensive Care Unit to a pediatric floor. She challenged the nurses on the child's diet, the frequency of treatments on the respirator, and his position in bed. When the child's nurse explained that she was following the doctor's orders and that she had confidence in him, the mother blurted out that she thought the nurses did not know what they were doing, and that she could not leave her son unprotected. At first the staff believed that she was reacting to the gravity of the child's condition, and to the fact that he no longer had the extraordinary attention which was given by the staff of the Intensive Care Unit.
>
> The relationship between the mother and nurses deteriorated further after Judd reported to his mother that the night nurse had awakened him to give him a sleeping medication. Mrs. B. was so agitated that she proceeded to inform anyone who would listen of the nurse's "bizarre" behavior. The head nurse asked this mother to withhold her judgment and her statements to visitors until the night nurse could be consulted about this alleged incident. This request was interpreted by both mother and son as a further insult to them. They summoned their pediatrician, who agreed with them that the nurse had acted irresponsibly. The pediatrician appeased her without considering the facts, and the impact it would have on interdisciplinary and staff-family relationships.

Thereafter, tension grew between Mrs. B. and the nurses, as did the nurses' anger with the medical staff. They requested intervention of the nursing mental health consultant. As the facts came to light, it was learned that the nurse did in fact awaken the child to take vital signs and to give him a treatment. She gave Judd sleeping medication when he complained that he was unable to fall asleep again. These facts only incensed Mrs. B. further. She pointed out, quite correctly (as was discovered) that her pediatrician had informed her that he had discontinued all treatments. Investigation disclosed that the pediatrician was giving verbal instruction to Mrs. B. while the surgeon was writing orders that did not coincide. Justifiably this mother was alarmed about inconsistencies and the lack of coordination of services.

The incident had a positive side: It led to administrative examination of the policies governing requests for consultation and to new methods for writing orders.

The participation of a mother in her child's care only brought to the surface what had been a basic problem in communication and interdisciplinary relationships. The staff can avoid this kind of conflict when they realize that both the automatic blaming, or support of one discipline by another, constitutes mismanagement of a problem. Every complaint, however minor, needs serious consideration; i.e., acknowledgement, acceptance of the feelings expressed and understanding of the basic issues. This does not imply agreement with the opinions stated. If these precepts are followed, staff conflict will create positive opportunities for role definition, mutual understanding, and pulling together.

Unfortunately, in too many institutions where the staff has not developed a cohesive, therapeutic atmosphere, programs of parent participation have been abruptly terminated. Preparation for parent participation takes time and the support and assistance of mental health professionals to deal with interpersonal and professional conflicts which always arise. Once a program becomes unmanageable, one can predict an immediate return to traditional methods of dealing with families; i.e., to eliminate them from the hospital environment.

VISITING AND SEPARATING

Where parent participation and rooming-in are not permitted, or in instances when families are unable to take advantage of facilities which are offered, the best alternative in managing separation anxiety in young children is by instituting lengthy and flexible visiting privileges.

Not too long ago, the idea that parent visiting was detrimental to children prevailed among medical personnel. The fact that apparently serene patients became difficult (i.e., by their screaming and inability to accept the departure of parents) gave evidence to support this view. Such management problems following visiting hours led to the practice of severely curtailing or prohibiting visitation in order to hasten the "settling" process.

Separation Anxiety

Actually, separation from parents in young children initiates a process described by Robertson which progresses from protest to despair to denial.[4] Characteristically in Phase 1, the child is restless, cries a great deal, looks eagerly toward sights and sounds which may indicate the presence of his parent; he may at this stage reject comforting by the staff. In Phase 2, the child makes fewer attempts to alter the environment; crying diminishes and apathy sets in. It is a mourning state which is frequently misinterpreted as a positive sign. With the onset of Phase 3, the child demonstrates interest in his surroundings and acceptance of separation. He may appear to have forgotten the parent altogether and allows her departure without complaint.

Research of the past 2 decades has taught professionals that "settling" was a false adjustment, easily reversed by the arrival of parents; that visiting did not cause the children's discontent, but rather exposed the distress which lay behind the calm exteriors.[5] Furthermore, the young child who eventually ceased to react negatively to infrequent visiting was showing an impaired relationship to his parents. Subsequently, evaluation of children suffering severe maternal deprivation demonstrated persistent, long-term manifestations of this deprivation—impaired trust leading to difficulties in establishing close relationships, distractibility, diminished intellectual functioning and self-centeredness.[6]

The Management of Separation Anxiety

For the newborn to 6-month group there is little separation anxiety, although it may be observed toward the end of this period. While a young baby can discriminate between mother and others, he also readily accepts substitutes as long as his need for food, warmth and human closeness are met and dependable routines for care are established. However, once the infant develops a strong attachment to his mother, substitute mothering cannot adequately compensate for her absence. This occurs at approximately 6 to 7 months.

The baby indicates displeasure when his mother is out of sight and rejects the attention of strangers. His reactions may range from minor episodes of crying to periods of terror. Young babies cannot understand, and will not learn for months to come, that objects continue to exist when they are out of sight. This fact poses a difficult problem when a parent is not available during hospitalization of an older infant.

Parents and staff need to work together to minimize the difficulties. Certainly frequent and regular visiting must be emphasized so that even in illness family relationships are maintained, and the parents' sense of adequacy in caring for their child is preserved. Staff responsibilities increase in the absence of a stable parent figure. Though frequent parental visits with their ensuing upsets cause difficulties of their own, they are worthwhile. The staff needs much support to tolerate the constant protest reactions of children. For babies there is a greater need for consistent assignment of personnel in order to develop trust (the anticipation that his needs will be met). (See Guidelines for Working with Infants, page 139.)

A baby will be less fearful of strangers when he is given opportunities to regard medical personnel as safe people. He responds well to an indirect approach; e.g., when the staff pays attention to others in his presence, works in his room away from his crib, and avoids making facial contortions and loud noises. Ideally, the baby will make the first overture for attention, indicating that the staff member is being accepted.

Babies can be helped by parents and staff to cope with separation anxiety through repetitive games in which people and objects appear and disappear.[7] Peek-a-boo serves this purpose as does hide-and-seek for toddlers. These games can also be initiated by the child. This "active mastery" brings presence and absence, under the child's control, and turns the unhappy, passive experience into a happy, playful occasion.

For toddlers, as well as for chidren under 4 years, sudden and prolonged separation can be overwhelming. Because these young children do not understand the concept of time, a few hours may seem like an eternity to them. These children can only be reassured by the actual presence of the parents. (See Guidelines for Working with Toddlers and Young Threes, page 141.) Beyond the age of 4, there is some understanding and anticipation of mother's return.

The amount of anxiety shown varies greatly with the individual child, depending upon his developmental level, the extent of his social contacts outside of the immediate family, and his former experiences with separation. Generally, the child with a strong and exclusive relationship with his mother will show the most severe reaction; those who do not have strong ties will have little to mourn and instead will form indiscriminate or close ties to the staff. (See story of Philip, page 216.) Naturally, most children in this age range are somewhere between these extremes.

The child's reactions need to be interpreted to parents as normal, acceptable, and the only way the child has of telling about his sorrow. The parents also need to realize that the child's grief can be lessened by a regular visiting pattern that can be described to him in terms of the sequence of ward activities, rather than setting the exact time that the parents will visit; e.g., "Mommy will be here after naptime tomorrow." The child will also be reassured if he is told that he is loved and that he will be going home again. These suggestions are most important for parents who stay away because they find the child's response too painful for them, or mistakenly believe that a subdued facade or rejection of them in favor of the staff indicates that they are not essential to the child. (See story of Jack, page 219.) Most children will find some comfort in keeping personal articles belonging to their parents and in showing family photos to the staff. Mother substitutes may be required for children whose parents visit irregularly.

As the child matures, his dependency needs decrease, and he is able to tolerate parental absence better. Although the school age child may still be lonely and homesick, he can find some comfort in peers and new interests. Evidence of separation anxiety is found in regressive tendencies, e.g., baby talk, petulance, irritability, bragging. Coping styles change: the older and more verbal the child, the less need he has to act out his feelings. The following examples indicate some of the foregoing age-specific reactions.

> Sean, age 3, had a gigantic tantrum on his mother's departure. Rallying, he sought the company of his favorite nurse whom he found in the nurses' station. She acknowledged his presence but indicated that she also was not free to be with him. Sean's rage was reactivated on being disappointed again. He proceeded to pull down his pants and "deposited" a large stool in the middle of the floor. His communication was direct and visible.

> Josh, age 6, confidently told his mother that she could leave him during his nap time. Once she was gone, he regretted his bravado. He buzzed the nurses' station and over the intercom told the staff in a quivering voice that his mother had just left and he needed to stay with someone right away. Fortunately, his

request was quickly fulfilled. When the incident was brought to the attention of his mother, and Josh was praised for his ability to communicate his needs, his mother said that she had advised her child that medical personnel were always on hand to help children, and that he could rely on them. This child had promptly put the information to a test. The favorable response to his request greatly influenced Josh's development of positive feelings toward the staff throughout his hospitalization.

ENCOUNTERS WITH PARENTS— TEACHING HOW TO PREPARE CHILDREN FOR HOSPITALIZATION

Most parents have given their child an initial explanation for hospitalization prior to admission. It is important to determine in the early family interview what has been said and how realistic a picture the child has received. Usually there is a need for correction or clarification according to the child's developmental level. However, the more difficult task is to deal with mothers and fathers who have been unable to tell their children that hospitalization is required, or who have gained their child's cooperation by deceit. (See also chapter on family.) This may be due to a variety of reasons—not the least of which are their own anxieties. Some parents believe that young children do not have the capacity to understand or to cope with the knowledge once it is given; others do not know what to say and abdicate responsibility altogether.

Professionals can help parents perform more adequately both before and after admission. When the staff finds that explanations are being withheld due to insufficient knowledge on the part of parents, it becomes obvious that the staff needs to play an active role earlier. This aspect of parental inadequacy can be easily remedied by the help of the personnel of clinics and by private pediatricians. Guidance and information can be dispensed verbally or in printed form. Two examples of the latter follow— *Preparing Your Child for Hospitalization and Eye Surgery* and *Preparing Your Child for Hospitalization and Tonsillectomy.*

Prospective patients should have a booklet that is specific for an institution, designed to acquaint the child with various aspects of hospital life in a nonthreatening fashion—taking into consideration physical structure, various personnel and their functions, equipment commonly used in caring for children and the daily routines. As substitutes, publications that accurately portray hospital activities in general would be acceptable.* A recent trend is the use of the pre-hospital visit as a preview of coming experiences. A variety of methods is valuable in introducing the subject of hospitalization as long as there is always opportunity for discussion. These methods are geared to increase a child's understanding and to present hospitalization as helping the child to get well. All these factors serve to minimize distorted ideas that lead to anxiety.

PREPARING YOUR CHILD FOR HOSPITALIZATION AND TONSILLECTOMY

Usually a first hospitalization is an unpleasant and frightening experience. The following steps can be taken to help you and your child understand the procedure and hospital routine; thereby making your child as comfortable as possible.

Some guidelines are proposed below which can help you answer your child's questions before he or she arrives at the hospital. We will carefully explain the admission procedure and preoperative routine to you and you will receive printed instructions as well.

Before admission, it is important that the child be told why he or she is going to the hospital and what is likely to happen while he is there. Once he is a patient, the medical and nursing staffs make every effort to explain procedures to both you and your child.

Children need to know that the tonsils are two little lumps in the back of the throat; that because the tonsils sometimes cause trouble (for instance: sore throats, ear aches or whatever symptoms common for your child) and are no longer needed; they are going to be removed. For this reason, he will be coming to the hospital to have an operation. Also tell him that no other part of the body will be operated upon.

Tell your child that he or she will be receiving a sweet-smelling medicine through a "space mask" which will keep him from feeling the operation. Afterward however, he will have a sore throat; he needs to know this. Tell him, too, that doctors and nurses know how to make his throat feel better and that in a few days he will be completely well.

For children between 4 and 7 years, it is a good idea to inform the opportunity to think about it and to ask questions. For very young them of the admission date 4 to 7 days in advance. This will give your child children, between 2 and 3 years, telling them 2 to 3 days before and on

---

* Examples are: Clark, B.: Pop-up Going to the Hospital. New York, Random House, 1970; Collier, J.: Danny Goes to the Hospital. New York, W. W. Norton, 1970; Rey, M., and Rey, H. A.: Curious George Goes to the Hospital. New York, Houghton Mifflin Co., 1966; Weber, A.: Elizabeth Get Well. New York, Thomas Y. Crowell, 1970.

the morning of admission is ample time. For children over 7, frank discussion a few weeks ahead and actual participation in the planning is advisable.

In order to help children discuss the coming operation, it is helpful for parents to ask simple questions to determine how much information the child has retained. For example: "Why do you have to have your tonsils out?" "Where are they?"

The younger the child, the more important it is for his mother to remain with him. Mothers are encouraged to stay with young children the day and night of surgery. When this is not possible, do not promise. When a parent is unable to stay with the child, we encourage her to be present before the child goes to the operating room and when he returns to the floor. Visiting hours are liberal. Your child should know when you are leaving and when you may be expected to return. Goodbyes may be difficult and tearful, but evasive answers only increase the child's anxiety and make him mistrust everyone. The emphasis should be on the certainty of your return.

To help your child understand hospitalization better, try reading some books to him concerning a hospital experience such as *A Visit to the Hospital* by Dr. Lester Coleman or *Curious George Goes to the Hospital* by Margaret and H. A. Rey. Also, allowing him to play with a doctor's kit may be helpful. Telling your child about your own experiences with hospitals, if they were fortuitous, is also anxiety relieving.

PREPARING YOUR CHILD FOR HOSPITALIZATION AND EYE SURGERY

Hospitalization is a new and often bewildering experience for a child, but careful preparation helps him to understand and accept necessary procedures. Because we know that parents frequently have questions regarding this preparation, we are proposing some guidelines for making this task easier for you.

Before admission, it is important that the child be told why he is going to the hospital and what is likely to happen when he gets there. Once he is a patient, the medical and nursing staffs will make every effort to explain procedures to him and his parents.

Your child needs to know that he is coming to the hospital because he has an eye condition which the doctor knows how to correct. Tell him he was born this way (if true); that you don't know why but no one is to blame. Often children think that their condition or hospitalization is a punishment. Make it clear to him that this is not so.

Try to explain his eye condition in terms of what he can visualize. For instance, if his eyes turn in or out too much, tell him that the doctor knows how to do an operation to make his eyes look straight so that he will look better. Tell him too, that he will be receiving some sweet-smelling medicine through a "space mask" which will keep him from feeling the operation or any hurt, and afterward, he will have a bandage on his eye (eyes) because the doctor will want his eye to rest for a while. After a day or so, he may go home. Also tell him that no other part of the body will be operated upon.

You have probably given your child some explanation of his eye condition in the past—for visits to the eye doctor, when his tests were given or when eye patches or glasses were used to treat his condition. At this time, it is helpful to remind your child of past explanations or treatments and to relate this new information to surgery.

It's a good idea to begin 4 to 7 days before admission if your child is 4 years or older, so that he will have time to think about it and ask questions. For very young children, between 2 and 3 years, telling them 2 to 3 days before and on the morning of admission is ample time. For children over 7, a frank discussion a few weeks ahead and actual participation in the planning is advisable.

In order to help your child discuss the coming operation, it is helpful for parents to ask simple questions to determine how much information the child has absorbed. For example: "Why do you have to have an eye operation?" or "What will you have on your eye afterward?" For the very young group, explanations can be given more easily by doll play—that is, pretending the doll is going to the hospital to have his eyes fixed and having your child put bandages or eye patches on the doll. We are constantly amazed at how much the child learns from this little drama.

The younger the child, the more important it is for the mother to remain with him. It is advisable for one parent to room in or to visit as much as possible. Visiting hours are liberal. Your child should know when you are leaving and when you may be expected to return. Good-byes may be difficult and tearful, but evasive answers only increase the child's anxiety and make him mistrust everyone.

In planning for hospitalization bring some familiar sounds from home—a musical toy or records and any toys or security objects to give him comfort. A doctor's kit is helpful both before and after a trip to the hospital. Try reading a book to him concerning a hospital experience such as *Curious George Goes to the Hospital* by M. and H. A. Rey.

When parents are encouraged to take the initial steps and are given the tools with which to do so, it is rare to find that they resist following through. However, the incidence of unprepared patients is still too high; thus, in addition to specific information regarding illness and treatment, the anxious and deceptive parents need to be told how detrimental their reactions are to the child's security. If they cannot change, then arrangements for parents to talk with a mental health specialist must precede further plans for the child.

Parent Participation in the Hospital Teaching Program

Once the child is admitted to a pediatric unit, responsibility for additional emotional preparation rests with the staff. Ideally, parents should participate in the stories, games, and explanations that help the child to anticipate and understand diagnostic, medical and surgical procedures. In order to do so, they require advance briefing so that they may employ the same principles and techniques used by medical personnel.

Whether or not parents actively participate in the preprocedural teaching, they must be cognizant of what the child has been told in order to be able to reinforce the kind of information the child receives. Clinical judgment needs to be made on how and when the parents are to be included. When parents demonstrate cooperative attitudes and are in control of their emotions, their presence during a teaching session can be beneficial for them and supportive for the child. However, when parents are obviously anxious or uncooperative, it is wise to exclude them from the instruction. In this case the child is likely to perceive the parents' anxiety or staff-parent conflict and associate this with the efforts to help him cope.

Occasionally parents are openly opposed to the psychological preparation of their children. One of the most frequent objections is to telling children so much. This might be a valid point if explanations were not geared to the needs of the individual child; that is, if "telling" was not related to age, family situation, illness, intellectual and emotional development. Parents need to know that whenever reasonable explanations concerning the nature of illness and treatment are absent or unclear, it is characteristic of the child to formulate his own conclusions about what is taking place as his way of coping with threats to his body. This often results in fantasies reflected in the child's current preoccupations. Distorted ideas if unclarified, may be more frightful than realistic presentations and can become obstacles to healthy emotional development. Clarification was possible in the following cases once the fantasies were disclosed.

Soon after 2-year-old Amy acquired a sibling, she was admitted to the hospital for repair of an umbilical hernia. She explained to her nurse that she was brought to the hospital because her mother did not want her anymore.

Mrs. K. refused to allow preoperative teaching for Douglas, age 3, who was hospitalized for repair of hypospadias. She thought that too much attention had been given to the congenital anomaly already, and she wanted to play down his problem. No amount of discussion deterred her from this position. On the day before surgery, Mrs. K. became enraged upon hearing from Douglas that his nurse had told him he was going to have his "pee pee" cut off. This statement was interpreted to the mother as her son's preoccupation and fear. The nurse again offered to explain events so that Douglas could be helped to understand, but Mrs. K. remained opposed. Hours later an evening nurse heard a similar tale—that a janitor told Douglas his penis would be cut off. The nurse was skeptical—explaining that it was the child's fantasy but she promised to investigate. On the following morning when Douglas reported that the dietitian told him that his penis would be taken off that day, it finally occurred to Mrs. K. that the child was asking for reassurance. She apologized to the staff and asked for help in preparing him for the operation.

After admitting Leo, age 5, for a cardiac catherization, Mrs. L. asked if there was anything she could do to make hospitalization less traumatic for her son. The nurse suggested that she reinforce the teaching repeatedly since children in Leo's age group were frequently fearful that other parts of the body might be involved in whatever procedure was described. "Oh," she said, "Now I know what that was all about. This morning as we were getting ready to come here, I saw Leo holding his penis in front of the mirror and saying to himself, I wonder what could be wrong with it.' "

When his nurse asked Keith, age 10, what he knew about undescended testicles and how they might have developed, he was quick to tell her the family myth. "I was dropped by my older sister when I was 2-months-old. That's when the testicles happened." It was suggested to him that although he had a complete physical examination after his sister dropped him, the problem had existed at birth. His response was, "She never liked me." The story was discussed with his mother who supported Keith's beliefs. She agreed that the incident was the basis of much of the anger which Keith harbored against his adolescent sister. Unwittingly the family had reinforced sibling hostilities and guilt in their children. They were surprised when they realized that the blame could not be put on anyone.

Will, age 7, developed visual disturbances and was hospitalized for diagnostic studies. His parents were so overwhelmed with the realistic possibility of brain tumor, they could not discuss the illness with him. Will told his nurse that he had figured out by himself that he was admitted to have his eyes removed.

Ruby, age 6, required periodic transfusions because of a rare congenital blood dyscrasia. After a particularly severe nasal hemorrhage, she told her nurse a story of a mother and father who placed candles around a coffin in their living room for a little girl who finally ran out of blood.

Jenny developed precocious puberty and an insatiable appetite at age 4 because of a brain tumor. She attributed these symptoms to a little man in her stomach who ate her food and caused her trouble.

Christina, age 4, was hospitalized for evaluation of adrenogenital syndrome. Her clitoris was quite prominent. Although this child spoke no English, her fantasy was clear enough. She frequently attempted to urinate in a standing position and was found in the boys' bathroom on numerous occasions. The older boys found her annoying and sought to keep her out.

Beth's mother reported that her 9-year-old daughter, who was admitted to the hospital after a large cabinet fell upon her, was adjusting exceedingy well after her ordeal—although she required diagnostic studies to rule out the possibility of a bladder injury, and was on complete bed rest. Mrs. L. jokingly said that Beth liked the attention, as did her younger sister who had a tonsillectomy two days before. However, she was startled, when Beth confided that she believed she might have caused the accident in order to be treated as well as her sister.

When parental cooperation is lacking, the staff will most likely make progress in obtaining consent for teaching if they focus first on the needs of parents. If the staff ignores the parents' wishes, there is a greater possibility of open hostilities, resistance to preventive programs, and greater stress on the child.

Charles, age 7, was scheduled for cardiac surgery. His cardiologist unwillingly agreed to the parents' conditions for treatment

—that the child remain unaware of what was happening to him. Otherwise they threatened to leave the hospital. Mr. and Mrs. Y. were determined to protect their son from the knowledge of coming events. They believed that they alone understood what was necessary to keep the boy alive. Charles was told that he was undergoing a yearly checkup as were the other patients. The father invented ludicrous stories to answer his son's questions regarding equipment and procedures he saw on the unit. Although the staff assured the parents that their wishes would be respected (while making it clear that they were not in agreement with the parents' management), the parents were still uncomfortable and guarded Charles day and night for fear that someone might divulge the secret.

The staff was reluctant to allow the child to undergo such a harrowing experience without first attempting to influence the parents' views. The approach decided upon was to support the parents' decisions but to inform them that they themselves required preoperative teaching in order to avoid the shock of Charles' postoperative appearance.

They were briefed in the same manner used for children—with drawings, dolls and miniature equipment. As the sessions proceeded, the parents became less antagonistic, asked intelligent questions and confessed that they had no idea of the complexity of the situation. The nurse interjected that Charles would also be surprised, and that it might be wise to prepare explanations in advance. Before long, the staff noticed that Charles had acquired a doll with a chest tube attached. Mr. Y. claimed that it was the only concession he would make.

Luckily for the boy, his operation had to be rescheduled in order to accommodate another patient who required emergency cardiac surgery. In the interim, the parents met a mother whose child had just been prepared for a similar procedure. She was lavish in her praise of the staff—complimenting them on their sensitivity to the needs of children and on the techniques they use to introduce traumatic events in advance as a way of enhancing a child's coping abilities. This chance meeting raised serious doubts in their minds concerning their approach. They were completely shaken soon after when Charles told his father that something monstrous was about to happen to him. The futility of pretense was obvious. Subsequently, Mr. Y. undertook the teaching assignment himself.

COUNSELING PARENTS

Extended visiting and parent participation in child care increases the probability that medical personnel will be called upon to discuss with families not only the illness of the child, but also various aspects of growth and development, and adjustment problems of the patient and his siblings. Frequent topics of concern include the preparation of children at home for the arrival of newborns, the presence of congenital anomalies, and the death of the hospitalized child. Parents also ask for advice in managing general behavior problems of hospitalized children after their discharge. They may also request help to reintegrate the child into family routines if the hospitalization has been lengthy.

Preparing a Sibling for the Arrival of Premature Twins

Mrs. G. was offered little hope for the live birth of twins. She had suffered numerous still births and miscarriages due to erythroblastosis. Against her husband's wishes she became pregnant for one last time. The pregnancy itself was difficult. Mr. G., who regarded the pregnancy as one more failure to be endured, did not give support to his wife and was openly hostile toward her. Polly, age 6, was their only child; Howard had died of leukemia a few months previously at age 8.

Much to the amazement of the family and medical personnel, Mrs. G. delivered living twins prematurely. It was an event that held little prospect for celebration. The boys were frail and required heroic measures to sustain life. Within a month, however, it became evident that the infants would survive. Mr. G. praised his wife's bravery and wisdom in the face of such odds. The parents bought clothes and toys and finally named the twins.

Eventually it occurred to the mother that because of the pessimism surrounding the birth and because she was immersed in the process of dealing with her own feelings, she had not discussed the existence of twins with her 6-year-old. Now she asked for help on how to proceed with the explanation. She could not believe that her daughter had any idea about what had occurred.

In anticipation of Polly's visit to the Premature Nursery (where sibling visiting is allowed behind a glass barrier), she was told about the babies and their need for hospitalization until they grew stronger and bigger.

When Polly arrived the occasion was used to evaluate her reactions and understanding of the events. She told the nurse who was nearby that she was waiting to see her twins. The nurse said that she knew a set of twins named Tim and Tom. Polly became quite excited saying "Thems the ones. They're mine." Thereafter she was easily engaged in conversation regarding their appearance, size and attitudes prevailing at home. "They thought I didn't know, but I heard mommy on the telephone; I sneaked out of bed to listen. Daddy was very mad at her." The description of what she expected to see was so accurate that the nurse wondered how she knew so much. Polly was eager to tell. "My friends at school didn't believe that we had babies because they aren't at home. So I took the pictures of wee babies to school (referring to a booklet given to Mrs. G. showing prematures in isolettes) and my teacher told us all about them. So everyone believed how little they were."

Thus, Mrs. G. was wrong in assuming that her daughter was unaware of her pregnancy. When questioned about her knowledge of reproduction, Polly claimed that she had known babies were coming because her mother had gotten fat. She was also proud to reveal the difference between boys and girls—explaining that she had seen her friend Johnny's "thing-a-ling." She accepted the genital differences between boys and girls, and rejected the idea that some children thought that girls had lost their "thing-a-lings." "Naw," she said, "girls are like their mommies."

Polly had learned from her mother that the infants required treatment for a blood disease. She was asked if she knew anyone else who had a blood problem; consequently this question led into a discussion of her dead brother. "Well Howie died; he bled a lot. He finally went (she gestured thumbs up)." When pressed for details she explained that he went up with the angels when he died. Polly believed that the infants had the same illness that Howie had. When this was clarified, and she was assured that no one else in the family was affected, Polly seemed more relaxed.

To check whether Polly felt responsible for the babies' illness and Howard's death,* aspects of sibling rivalry were touched on. She was told a story about Henry, a boy who sometimes liked his baby brother and sometimes really hated him. When the baby was cute and wanted to play, he was fun; when the baby cried and took so much of mother's time, Henry did not want him to be part of the family. When Henry could not have his mother to himself, he was jealous and had some pretty bad thoughts—he

* This is egocentric thinking. Children under 6 normally think this way; older children sometimes do, i.e., in terms of the world revolving around them and with things happening because of their personal actions.

wanted to get rid of that baby. This boy was just like everybody else—sometimes he loved a person, and sometimes he did not. When the baby became sick, Henry got the idea that the baby was sick because he had wished it. This boy did not know that you can not harm people by thoughts. Polly's response indicated that she understood quite well and experienced some guilt at her own wish to be rid of rivals. Soon after she allayed her guilt by saying, "Aw, wishes never come true."

Happily, it was possible to report to Mrs. G. that Polly was coping exceptionally well, and that it was a tribute to her parents that this was true. Although their current crisis had temporarily overtaxed Mr. and Mrs. G.'s capacity to deal with their daughter's needs, it was obvious that Polly's straight thinking, extensive verbal abilities, and skill in obtaining the help she wanted indicated a solid child-parent relationship and good family adjustment.

The parents were advised to convey to Polly the fact that all subjects were open to discussion—especially sibling rivalry; to encourage her to express her thoughts about the twins and her dead brother; to assure her that nothing she could imagine or think would eliminate her special place in the family.

Experience with this mother showed the staff that under pressure she resorted to massive denial of reality, and that in future hospitalizations of her children, she might once again do so. Many women use this mechanism to cope with feelings about exceptional children.

Explaining Congenital Anomaly

A question frequently raised is the advisability of telling the siblings of the hospitalized child about illness or obvious congenital anomalies—whether explanations are in order and what to say. A significant point to consider is that children always come to some conclusions on their own whenever information is withheld. These conclusions are usually erroneous and painful to endure. With diplomatic assistance, most parents can be helped to present the facts with words appropriate to the child's emotional and intellectual level while offering reassurance at the same time.

Mrs. R. did a creditable job in preparing her 3½-year-old daughter for the arrival of a sister. (See explaining sibling rivalry to Polly.) However, the homecoming was delayed when the newborn developed a bowel obstruction which required a colostomy. Although the parents wanted to present a factual picture to their older child, they hesitated in discussing the subject, thinking it was too complex for her to understand. They were relieved to hear that a simple explanation was possible and suitable. The parents told Annie that after her sister was born, she had trouble making "do do" from her "coolie" (parent's jargon), and that the doctors had helped her by making a small opening on her belly for the "do do" to come out. They also told her that eventually the doctors could fix it so that she could make "do do" from below. She was told that no one knew why the baby was born that way, but that no one was to blame. (See *Egocentric thinking,* page 23.) Because the mother was admitted shortly after to a neighboring hospital for a hysterectomy, the father was asked to further reassure Annie that she was not going to be the next one to have an opening made in the tummy, nor was he.

Helping Parents to Prepare Siblings for the Death of a Child

Because the subject of death arouses painful emotions in all people, it is often avoided where it needs to be discussed the most. Medical personnel have difficulty with this topic and hesitate to discuss with parents how they are coping with terminal illness and what arrangements have been made to prepare the other children. Death is an unavoidable issue in which all pediatric staff will eventually become involved. Advance planning allows the staff to be of greater assistance to parents and to deal more confidently with this emotionally charged area. (See Chapter 7.)

Surprisingly, though all too frequently, siblings at home are expected to manage on their own. Professionals need to introduce the subject of how the children at home are affected by the illness, what questions they ask, and what answers they get during the parents' long absences. This would reveal that even with the milder experiences of long separations, explanations to siblings are inadequate since these children are not totally ignorant of what is happening around them. Children are seldom completely in the dark. Even a very young child senses a change in mood or picks up anxiety. Silence itself can have a foreboding, ominous quality. In these circumstances, children who are not informed about separation will be left to bear the complete burden of dealing with these complex feelings. Families who deal poorly with separation also mismanage the more final loss—death.

Children deserve an explanation, but many parents fear that a discussion of illness and impending death would break down their own controls, and lead to their own disintegration. Hence these parents assume that their children would be likewise beset, and so they keep silent. Parents need reassurance that exposure of their feelings would reveal that they care and have the strength to feel deep compassion. They need to be told that children have the strength to withstand grief reactions. This may come as a surprise to many adults who have a pollyanna view of childhood.

When children are allowed to hear their parents openly discussing their hopes and concerns about the sick child, they too should be given permission to participate. They may take the opportunity to ask questions about the nature of the illness and treatment. In the absence of questions, information can be interjected by the parents. After initial talks, parents are then ready to comment on the possibility that the patient may not get well despite all that is being done, and later on that he is not expected to live. When there is adequate time, this explanation can be carried out gradually.

Children of all ages could and do tolerate the witnessing of a very sick sibling. The total impact obviously depends on the child's understanding, the reactions of the adults, and the constancy of the parents' support of the sibling.

After the child has died, the parents should not tell the remaining children to remember the deceased as he was in the fullest bloom of life. This statement would cause the children to believe that life is tenuous and can easily end despite good health. On the other hand, the sudden viewing of a dead body without foreknowing that the grown-ups may be upset, can cause the children to have a lasting painful memory of seeing an immobile, dead figure.

Discussions before death occurs allow siblings to make amends for their hostilities toward the sick child. Ambivalence in families is usual. Children need to come to grips with both positive and negative feelings about the sick child and need to know that each is acceptable. A sick child in any family is quite an irritant, usually causing short or long-term neglect of the siblings by parents and requiring much sacrifice in finances and mobility. It is only natural for siblings to wish that the sick child either be well or dead. They may also welcome the idea of performing small acts of kindness before death—visiting, sending gifts and writing letters.

Mrs. H. accompanied her 8-year-old to the hospital in the terminal stages of his illness. During 10 weeks of rooming-in, she won the respect of the staff who was constantly impressed by her stoicism. However, her courage failed her temporarily after Matthew was placed in protective isolation. The isolation made it difficult for her to take frequent, small breaks from his bedside because of the inconvenience of washing, masking and gowning. Consequently, she remained with Matthew for long, uninterrupted periods and found the tension unbearable.

On one occasion Mrs. H. ran out into the hallway in tears, asking to talk to someone. She explained that she feared losing control in Matt's presence and that her feelings of grief were so intense she could not hide them from him. The staff took the opportunity to discuss with her what she believed Matt knew about his illness. She sincerely thought that he had no knowledge of the seriousness of his condition, and that she had succeeded in protecting him. However, the fact that she and Matt had become more and more withdrawn from one another indicated otherwise. (See Chapter 7.) Her reactions were observed. Because she could not discuss her preoccupations with Matt, she did not communicate with him at all. It was suggested that if she broke down again, she should tell him that it was because she was sad about his sickness, and that sometimes she became discouraged and upset. Mrs. H.'s pretense that she was not sad, only denied the child's perceptions and made it impossible for him to confide in her and assuage his own anxieties.

On the same occasion Mrs. H. discussed with the nurse, the reactions of other members of the family. Her husband was her main support, but he was not available because they lived a distance from the hospital. He was caring for their 2 sons with the assistance of several neighbors who took turns inviting them for meals. Mrs. H. confided that she and her husband were unable to be truthful with the older children fearing that if they were aware of impending death for a long period of time, they might become insecure. The possibility was mentioned of her visiting the boys over the weekend in order to prepare them for Matt's death, and in order to find a housekeeper so that the family could maintain a semblance of normal living. It made sense to her.

A few surprises awaited Mrs. H. on her arrival home. Both boys were quite aware of their brother's condition. The older boy disclosed that he had embarked on a project of scientific inquiry. His science teacher directed the class to investigate a problem by collecting data, discarding the irrelevant material and coming to a conclusion on the basis of facts. Twelve-year-old Steven decided to research his brother's illness. His conclusion—leukemia.

Ten-year-old Luke's response to his brother's hospitalization was massive regression—demonstrated by clinging behavior, soiling, enuresis and learning difficulty.

Mr. H. was coping poorly. He found the questions the 2 boys asked about Matthew harassing because he was trying to divulge as little information as possible. Disorganization in the household led to his quick consent to acquiring a housekeeper.

On her return to the hospital Mrs. H. was eager to recount her experiences. In particular she wanted to find psychiatric help for Luke whose regression in this crisis gave impetus to her wish to have him see a professional. She was able to disregard what the anti-psychiatry neighbors would think. She said that something constructive had to come of this ordeal—and helping Luke would be it.

Mrs. H. tried a different approach with Matt. Instead of leaving his room the next time she was tearful she stayed, and a big teardrop fell on Matt's hand. He kidded her saying, "You're pretty sloppy in your old age Mom." Because of this response they were able to laugh, talk again, and cry together. Before long, Matthew was telling his mother that he was worried about himself too.

Preparing Parents for Discharge of the Child

Generally, a prediction of a child's posthospital adjustment can be made on the following criteria: the kind of preparation received before and during hospitalization, the extent of family involvement and support, the degree of emotional health prior to illness, and the adaptation made in the pediatric unit. The length of the hospital stay may be a factor, but not necessarily so; long-term illness can be a maturing experience for the patient whose management has been ideal; while, on the other hand, short-term illness may be devastating for the child whose developmental needs have not been considered. Gross behavioral disturbance, present before admission, or emerging under the stress of illness and treatment, can hardly be missed and will most likely require evaluation on an inpatient basis and professional follow-up. (See stories of Robinson, Whitney, Jill and Angela, Chapter 8.) As a rule the more subtle reactions do not command such specific attention. Nevertheless, parents need help in coping with them.

Conferences with families regarding physical care and convalescence present excellent opportunities for the staff to interject comments and suggestions that further the emotional well-being of children. Personnel who have had the greatest contact with the family and who have worked directly in helping the child with his feelings during hospitalization, are in the best position to counsel parents in preparation for the kinds of behavior seen so frequently at home. They need to know that phobias, nightmares, regression, negativism, and disturbances in eating and learning are common aftermaths of hospitalization and indicate unresolved difficulties.

Suggestions to Staff

At the onset of the conference it is important to give parents support by acknowledging their distress and courageous behavior during the child's illness, and then by expressing confidence in their ability to cope with problem situations. This praise can be elaborated upon when hospitalization has been lengthy and parents have responded well to the crisis. In instances where the parents have not responded well, an expression of understanding the parents' circumstances is necessary but insufficient. These parents then need to be given a list of behavioral danger signals that require a return to professionals for help and guidance.

When problem behavior in the child is demonstrated before discharge (e.g., eating or disciplinary problems), the staff can indicate to the parents what measures they have taken and how parents can participate in the plan. Any practice they have with influencing behavioral change in their child is reassuring to the many who are skeptical of this program. Parents may come to realize that difficulties developing after discharge are the residual effects of hospitalization. While this knowledge may make them more tolerant of clinging, loss of recently acquired skills (bowel and bladder control), revengeful attitudes, or fears of strangers, this does not imply that these manifestations should be passively tolerated. Parents' confidence is buttressed when they are supplied with guidelines for the management of regression. They can:

1. Return the child to integrated family life as soon as possible. This means giving the child the responsibilities equal to his abilities.

2. Acknowledge the child's bravery but refrain from making him the center of attention because of sickness. There is danger in his using symptoms for attention (secondary gains). Lots of hugs and kisses can be lavished when the hospital "veteran" does something cute or constructive, but unrelated to his illness. Include pleasurable activities in his routines.

3. Be kind, firm, and consistent especially in the management of disciplinary problems.

4. Be truthful in order to preserve a child's trust.

5. Provide play materials such as clay, paints, doctor and nurse kits, and equipment given to him in the hospital. Allow the child to play on his own.

6. Permit the verbal child to express his feelings regarding illness and

hospitalization. Clarify distortions in his understanding. This expression of feelings helps the child to integrate experiences into his life rather than to deny them.

7. Avoid leaving the child for long periods or overnight until he is well adjusted and trusting of his safety at home.

8. Allow the child to visit the staff in between admissions, when in the hospital vicinity or after clinic appointments.

Suggestions Particular to Parents of Children With Congenital Anomalies and Exceptional Children

Parents of children with congenital anomalies need the long-term support and counseling from the member of the health team whom they know best—physician, nurse, social worker. Too often, the parents are so preoccupied with the child's adjustment to adulthood that they exclude giving attention to his contemporary adaptation. A change from their focussing on the long range goals (which may be revised in the light of new knowledge) to appropriate age developmental tasks—trust, autonomy, initiative, is required to minimize the additional emotional difficulties common for handicapped children. This change in approach frequently depends upon the parents' resolution of anxiety related to the birth of an exceptional child. Anxiety causes these parents to deny the immediate emotional impact by concentrating on the future, but the price is too high. Such a child would never develop skills leading to mature behavior. Other parents use of egocentric thinking can cause them increased guilt. They place blame on themselves or project this blame onto a spouse.

> Mrs. W. explained her toddler's congenital heart defect in relation to "bad thoughts" during her pregnancy. Her husband agreed with her.

> Mrs. F. regularly claimed her family to be free of blood diseases, so that her child's blood disease had to come from her husband's side of the family.

Although these parents need the utmost of compassion, the mental health team should encourage all staff members to avoid the pitfall of oversolicitous reinforcement of parental self-pity. The parental marriage may be strained by the birth of an abnormal child. Only through the total assessment of the family can staff members know when to intervene between parents who have started to drift apart. There is a discrepancy between what the parents expected and what they got. The reality contrasts unfavorably with the ideal image, which leads to disappointment and anger. Parents are then, often guilty about this wish to be rid of the strange child before them. This dynamic, universal, and normal reaction must be explored and explained as normal before parents can be told of modern science's ways of helping the child overcome his inborn deficiencies. They need to be helped to mourn the loss of the perfect child "that might have been."

ROUNDS

Scrutiny of medical and nursing rounds will reveal in most instances that they are oriented to sickness in children rather than to children who are sick. This happens in any hospital where there is the tradition of combining 2 major functions simultaneously: staff education and assessment of patient progress. Understanding the effects of this practice on children may lead to more constructive ways of implementing each of these equally important functions. Any change in the way rounds are conducted requires advance agreement on the purpose of rounds, the implementation of the rounds, and the advocacy of the mental health team. The first practical outcome of change is for all discussion to take place in a location that respects both the child's right of not being in the position to overhear, and the professional right to confer in quiet, orderly dignity.

Much of the distorted information patients and parents obtain comes by way of careless remarks and eavesdropping during rounds.

> Eric, age 4, overheard his doctors discussing arrangements for a bone marrow aspiration. After overhearing this he asked his mother if he was to have a bow and arrow.

> At 15, Carol, a sophisticated and knowledgeable adolescent who was admitted for the treatment of subacute bacterial endocarditis quickly lost her facade when she heard the pediatricians discussing the mortality rates for her disease.

> Jane's examining physician casually mentioned that she could not feel the child's ovaries. Not until much later did the staff learn from her father that this 13-year-old had interpreted the statement to mean that she had no ovaries.

Nancy, age 10, was quite depressed as a result of several setbacks following cardiac surgery. Her feelings of hopelessness were reinforced when, during rounds, her pediatrician said in an effort to be reassuring, "Well, there is nothing more we can do for you." Her anxious expression was picked up by the head nurse who explained that the doctor meant to say all the diagnostic tests he had ordered were already carried out.

Fourteen-year-old Carrie's anxious parents were present in the Intensive Care Unit when a surgeon checking the child's condition said to the nurse as he was making adjustments, "There is too much negative pressure in the chest tube." The parents became convinced that an error was made and that their child was incompetently managed.

A child who is hospitalized for the first time needs a special briefing on the meaning of rounds. Having a group of people surround his bed can be a frightening experience until he learns that it is routine procedure for doctors to see how each child is progressing. He needs to know that he will be examined by several people in addition to his own doctor, and that often there will be strangers who join the staff on their rounds. Naturally, the child would expect to be introduced. Parents, if included in this briefing, can repeat this explanation to their child so his understanding is clearer.

Although effective rounds should have a give and take quality between the patient and rounder, this is unlikely to occur unless the child feels safe enough to speak up. It helps to make personalized statements such as: "It's not easy for you to be here"; "I guess we interrupted your T.V. program"; "It's nice to see you again though I wish it were outside the hospital"; "We'll try not to take too long." In other words the patients should be included in the rounds rather than being made specimens that are observed "under glass."

A common error of many professionals who have had limited contact with children, is to be ebullient, overly familiar, and coy. Sometimes the child is encouraged to call staff members by their first names. Although this first-name style of addressing the doctor might be appropriate for older children in certain cases, it is safer to assume that first names confuse the child; he believes that he can control the adult professionals, when in fact he has very little authority as an inpatient. What purpose first-name addressing serves the professional can only be guessed at. Young professionals may think that the adulation of a child confirms their clinical skills. The child ultimately suffers because the allure of a close tie to an older, powerful figure on the ward causes him to have expectations that cannot be gratified. The professional's time exigencies and lack of a personal attachment to this child can result in disappointment for the child. This buddy approach encourages the child to test the limits of the new and unfamiliar relationship, often to the surprise of the professional who cannot handle the child's brashness. To trifle with a child in this manner complicates his adaptation to the hospital.

> A medical student introduced himself to 8-year-old Billy, "I'm Jack," and continued, "I'm going to be examining and talking to you over the next few days." They told jokes together; Billy went through Jack's pockets. Within a few hours, Jack was being trailed by Billy who was shooting him with his favorite water-filled syringe, and shouting, "Hey Jack, come play!" The student asked his preceptor why he was having so much difficulty in enlisting the child's cooperation for any procedure. He complained of Billy's obstreperous and annoying antics. The preceptor, who knew Billy vaguely, advised the student to be very firm and to take the syringe from Billy. When this was done, Billy became quieter, but at the same time he muttered about his brother's strength to all who would listen.

Having considered the danger of overfamiliarity, and the need for orientation and circumspection in talk at the bedside, other common issues can be considered, such as the avoidance of giving the child the impression that he has a choice during the physical examination when there is in fact no choice. It is insincere to say, "May I listen to your chest?" when the child has been kept waiting for rounds, and 4 people have their stethoscopes ready. It is better to say "We are going to listen to your chest." Also, allowing the child to stall a part of the examination, as with the partial obstruction of any procedure, only makes the child more anxious. It is best to proceed firmly with the examination and get it over with. Talking to the child while the examination is going on helps to humanize the process, so that the child is not treated as an inanimate object. He needs to know in a simple way, what the doctors are looking for and what they have found. A child who is fearful of instruments might be allowed to play with one before it is used on him.

When the child is too young to understand what the doctors are discovering on the rounds, he can be told "You may not understand what is happening here; we will tell your mother who will explain to you later on what we're planning to do." An older child can be told "You can tell your parents that we're going to be doing _____," and "We'll be talking to them ourselves."

Children constantly think about what the rounds evaluation means so far as the possibility of their going home. It is better to keep this in mind and give them a rough idea of how long they will have to stay, rather than allowing them to think that the least improvement implies that they will be leaving the hospital; or contrariwise, that a new finding or procedure means their stay is to be prolonged.

Any grouping of beds in a unit should always be considered a dynamic environment; that is, when the staff tarries at the bedside of one child, the other children will wonder why he is getting special attention. The staff should explain that time spent by them at rounds has no relation to whether or not that child being considered has been bad or good, is liked more, or is getting better or worse. Rather the children should know that the time spent with a child is related to whether he has just arrived, if he needs extra attention to get to know him or if he has to have a new series of treatments. They should also know that those children who are completely passed by are not forgotten and neglected but are unchanged or progressing uneventfully; thus they do not need medical work. These "passed by" children need to be encouraged to say if they are disappointed when someone on rounds does not say hello.

Then there is the child who is seen a second time by a few professionals after rounds are over because he has an interesting physical sign they wish to study. For this child, the rounds begin again, creating all the foregoing concerns in others who are in that unit. It also calls too much attention to the child's body, almost implying that now that he is sick, he has something of value. Unless absolutely necessary, this "doubling back" should be limited and carefully presented to the child in order to minimize these effects. Children may regard the rounds as an unnecessary intrusion on their activities. In their beds quiet children may give no hint of their deeper feeling about a group of adults who invade the privacy of their bodies with hands and instruments. Also these grown-ups utter large words, snatches of which are easily distorted.

Periodically, there are larger rounds on the floor; then the atmosphere becomes more austere and the expectations greater for the child to behave. These special rounds usually interfere with daily routines. Older children should be dispatched as soon as possible to respect their privacy and to free them for activities. Younger children can tolerate waiting in their beds as they are there anyway. Efforts should be made to ensure that even these rounds are for the benefit of the child and not merely to use him as a curiosity.

Rounds create an occasion for staff dissension. Doctors who are disease-oriented and short of time may be self-absorbed and unaware of the commotion they cause as they enter the scene. Parents, when present, solicit and welcome all the attention and reassurance they can get during rounds, and this could easily cause their demands to annoy the staff.

Another possible source of conflict within the staff is that orders for the care of children are written which affect non-physician professionals such as play therapists, teachers, and social workers. In the mildly hectic atmosphere of rounds, these staff members rarely have the opportunity to contribute their experience. Other staff members who are not present at rounds will be instructed to treat the child without participating in these decisions. This built-in conflict is so obvious that it is one of the earliest areas of mental health team intervention in order to assure smooth functioning of professional groups.

One way to ameliorate this problem is to have the paramedical personnel on the staff regularly write notes in the medical chart. This information then could be included as part of the complete daily picture of each child. The mental health team serves to encourage all professionals to speak up if their documented work is ignored.

If the doctor's rounds approach the above ideal, it is likely that emotional disorders will be picked up for consultation at earlier phases of hospitalization. Furthermore, certain medical and surgical procedures could be easily modified in the light of individual needs; thus combining both the physical and emotional.

Once conflict is diminished on rounds, it might be possible to see this modification reflected in the furthering of each child's development. Rounds would then need to chronicle daily the atmosphere of each grouping of children, and the floor as a whole. (When this is achieved, the mental health team can recede in its activities.) Because isolated needs of children are taken care of in separate ways, the maximum promotion of health in children requires the coordination of the total environment.

THE ROLE OF THE LIAISON PSYCHIATRIST

The psychiatrist who works with children in a pediatric setting can function in a variety of ways. One of the most effective ways is to integrate the traditional (liaison) consultation with primary and secondary prevention techniques.* These are applied to the population of staff, patients and families.

Often in the customary approach, the psychiatrist dismissed a healthy child as one who did not need any individual attention for coping with the crisis of illness, or for utilizing the hospital experience for furthering his maturation. Also traditionally, the psychiatrist alarmed the staff with jargon and ominous pronouncements. Psychiatric workers were seldom aware that their words had the power to create anxiety among the staff and families. Psychiatrists should try to limit their use of complex terminology which confuses, upsets, and intimidates the staff and the families.

In the customary approach, the usual service rendered was a psychiatric diagnosis based on data obtained from staff, parents and child. This diagnosis was a description given in a pathology-oriented context. Based on this description, a plan would be made that was individualized and limited to the disturbed.

In a more progressive program a psychiatrist provides the opportunity for staff development—to learn interview technique, play diagnosis, and methods for establishing rapport with difficult parents and children. He fosters a team approach to observations, teaches how to discard the irrelevant, and recalls similar problems and cases so that the staff can make connections with other examples of the same type. In this way generalizations are built up from clinical experiences. The psychiatrist shows how to make comprehensive assessments of family units and their interactions with the hospital environment.

Weekly rounds, led by this consultant with representatives from each discipline, can be an invaluable asset to maintaining the unified group approach. These discussions provide opportunities for teaching about children's reactions to illness. Establishing organized thinking about patient adjustment leads to practical programs of management and rapid evaluation of the child's status.

The psychiatrist (or mental health worker) can give to a child and his family a sense of continued relationship with a medical person who does not cause him pain (does not wear a white uniform) and who tries to focus on the child's point of view. Although the staff may emphasize the

---

* Primary prevention is "intervention in order to lower the risk of the child's becoming ill."
Secondary prevention is "prevention of the disability or a disorder through early and adequate treatment."

surface behavior (e.g., that unless the child takes in 'x' quantity of calories and fluid, he will physically deteriorate) the psychiatrist directs the staffs' thinking to underlying factors which could either cause or exacerbate the external behavior. In these ways the child and the staff are both directed toward treating the whole child.

When this program is fully institutionalized and with staff constancy, there is the opportunity to teach advanced concepts; such as, the existence of unconscious mechanisms, lifelong personality characteristics (habitual defensive patterns that exist in every person), and emergency reactions common to illness and separation.

In essence, the statement above is a job description for the psychiatrist that should be expected by the pediatric staff and supplied by the psychiatry department.

When the psychiatrist mistakenly assumes he is the only one knowledgeable—the team leader and final authority—other members on the staff do not feel useful. He needs to show an openness to the contribution of all personnel—nursing, social service, aides, interns, residents, attendants, recreation workers. The psychiatrist's limited contact with patients and parents compared with that of the staff, indicates that his most effective role is to rely on the latter's contributions rather than supplying and imposing his own ideas. For example:

> Mark, age 9, had a history of minor complaints as an attention-getting mechanism. The psychiatrist said to the resident pediatrician, "You handled that very well when you paid attention to the child's minor finger cut and put on the band-aid yourself, establishing a relationship with Mark that allowed him to sound off. This child obviously had ideas he wanted to express but required you to pass the test of handling the cut seriously."

The psychiatrist is steeped in his own field and should not use shorthand formulations and abstractions when working in another specialty. He is not there to confound the staff with his psychiatric jargon, but to show his usefulness and to encourage the staff to use their own talents for making children healthy.

The psychiatrist functions better as part of a mental health team than as an individual. Unless he spends his entire time in the nonpsychiatric field, he needs the follow-through and feedback from the personnel that are there continuously. For their part the personnel need to have absorbed enough of the psychiatric approach to utilize the psychiatrist's time most effectively and to have effective meetings without him. It would be wasteful if the psychiatrist had to decide who would or would not be brought before the staff for their in-service training.

The image of the psychiatrist needs to be clarified. He is generally viewed as permissive with the expectation that he will ask the staff to tolerate antisocial behavior—bad manners, sex play. The staff suppress their anger, thinking that the psychiatrist expects them to permit brashness. In fact, the psychiatrist is on the side of reasonable limit-setting to help pediatric workers do their jobs and also to reassure the children that adults are able to stop them if they lose control.

The psychiatrist contributes directly to professional staff development by teaching psychopathology and psychiatric treatment of special problems such as the antisocial, psychotic, and withdrawn child. There is also a need to teach the pediatrician how to do a competent mental status examination, and to know the indications for psychiatric consultation; e.g., depression, threat of suicide, withdrawal, bizarre behavior, gender identity problems, hyperactivity, certain precocities, etc. The integration of information from psychological testing is more conclusive when set in the context of staff assessment and total family evaluation. Furthermore, most children are in a stressful situation while in the hospital, and their performance on testing will reflect this stress by showing regression. A larger grasp of their adaptation to the environment is needed to arrive at an individualized treatment plan.

The cognitive information gathered from psychological testing can be compared to expected norms for that age and family type. (See Chapter 2.) Certain test responses can give a precise account of the particular symbols that continually threaten a child. For instance:

... Abandonment and death themes in a child who ended animal stories with the dog being left alone, or the bird losing its way down a cold, dark passage.

... Deprivation themes in a child who visualized snow hiding the food.

... Castration themes in a child who visualized fallen trees and smokestacks, damaged motors, and explosions.

The psychiatrist needs to avoid the psychopathological model that labels as disturbed, all strong reactions of sick children. What needs to be demonstrated to pediatric personnel is the tremendous human variability and wealth of behavior patterns which can be supported, modified, or altered to promote greater resiliency, adaptability, and ultimate strength. The art of medical management has always addressed itself to these ends, but with increasing specialization and scientific complexity, much of this art has been left by default to the psychiatrist.

The psychiatrist can humanize his own field by revealing the difficulties and removing the omnipotence and clairvoyance that other disciplines imagine. The purpose is not to convert pediatricians into psychiatrists, but to allow pediatric professionals to enrich their training with greater understanding of humans. Much of the knowledge psychiatry has to offer can be taught once the self-consciousness common to people who are exposed to it for the first time is overcome.

Working with sick children stirs up feelings which cause discomfort, thus impeding emotional availability. The psychiatrist can discern this. There is a need in these settings for people to meet, to support each other, and to share experiences so they can return to the wards and maintain an optimal attitude toward their small charges. In their different reactions to discomfort, staff disagreements may need the expertise of a psychiatrist's intervention.

Problems in Liaison Work

Psychiatry tends to arouse extremes of feelings. On the positive side there is the danger of oversell, wherein the staff becomes so expressive and emotional about their newfound and accepted feelings that floor conferences evolve into group therapy sessions where professionals "psych" each other. Every patient becomes a mental catastrophe, or the staff vies with each other to please and gain personalized attention from the psychiatrist.

On the negative side, pediatric personnel may come to reject psychiatric concepts completely. When a psychiatrist is critical, his words carry greater weight than intended because they are uttered by a mental expert. Hostile staff feelings rapidly generate without an intermediate person—a pediatrician interested in psychology, or a nursing mental health consultant, or a head nurse with special growth and development training to neutralize the criticism at its source or modulate the reaction.

> The psychiatrist wondered whether Nurse F. had not been too harsh in removing Andy's syringe when he squirted it. She was hurt but did not defend herself. Only later did the head nurse who missed the conference, take issue with the psychiatrist and explain that Andy had been kindly and repeatedly told not to use the syringe for that purpose. The next mental health conference raised the issue of staff reticence to defend themselves, and staff

deference in asserting themselves to the psychiatrist. It emerged that they feared his criticism.

Negative reactions are also evoked when there is a lack of common courtesies such as late arrivals, lack of clear recommendations, exaggerations, and lack of seriousness. The constructive approach for dealing with this is for the psychiatrist to have a continuous evaluation of his effectiveness. This can be done by soliciting the opinions of paramedical and administrative medical staff. The responsibility also rests with the pediatric department to spontaneously and regularly offer support and suggestions to the psychiatrist. Administrative acceptance is crucial to maintain a positive atmosphere about the value of liaison work. This is the only counterbalance at times of extreme resistance that can seriously impair the environmental program. (See Chapter 1.)

Of the two extremes, positive attitudes are more difficult to manage once they have developed. The psychiatrist is tempted to enjoy having friends among the pediatric staff. These friendships can easily lead to the development of favoritism and rivalry for his attention. He needs to treat the entire staff as an entity. Those individuals who single themselves out by confidentially relaying information to the psychiatrist that illuminates a facet of the child's personality, have to be skillfully shown how their observations and comments would benefit their colleagues.

Another delicate situation occurs when the staff utilize the psychiatrist for their own therapy. The staff member has to be given credence and assistance in his personal concern while gently being referred to the appropriate facility if indicated. At the same time, this person's work may be compromised by the personal issue expressed. The psychiatrist needs all his diplomacy to support this professional's continued effectiveness.

People working in academic settings are often highly competitive and at times are under stresses not apparent to transient consultants. The latter can be drawn into internecine battles and unwittingly enlisted to give recognition or take sides in a power struggle. For example:

Max's outside pediatrician sent him in for evaluation. Although he was reluctant to diagnose Max's grossly antisocial personality, he assumed that his difficult patient would be taken care of by the resource people. The pediatric resident found nothing medically treatable. Though Max's behavior was unremarkable for a 10-year-old, a radical change occurred when he was interviewed by the psychiatrist, who was trying to reveal the boy's basic personality and to expose the problem to the staff. The psychiatrist wanted to familiarize the staff with this kind of personality and to prepare them for managing the inevitable emergency situation that could develop without warning.

Max refused to talk, rapidly became abusive, and ran out of the room returning to throw a hot teapot onto the conferees. Nurses claimed that they wanted protection from him, and the psychology intern insinuated that psychiatry was stirring up the patients. On investigation, nursing took advantage of the incident to request more staffing; pediatric residents criticized the outside doctor for an unnecessary admission, and the psychology intern reasserted his plan to suppress the patient's emotions. Thus, each of the three groups used the patient's behavior to their own ends.

The care of any individual patient is then a coming together of many interests, and the challenge that it offers the psychiatrist may explain the fascination this work has for some.

The psychiatrist can promote the establishment of a team consisting of himself, the mental health consultant nurse, a psychiatric resident interested in liaison work, a pediatric resident taking a fellowship in child psychiatry, a clinical psychologist, a social worker, and a recreation worker.

The success of such an enterprise might be demonstrated by the ability of the pediatric staff to characterize each child individually, as part of a family and a culture. The nurses would know the ability of the child and his environment to cope with the stresses of life; e.g., the effect of this illness. The administration would understand that certain problems in children because of their complexity would create conflicts between departments. People in medicine and surgery, nursing, pediatrics and psychology, who usually vie to a greater or lesser degree for the child's time, might now synchronize their skills.

The ultimate success is signified by each pediatric floor operating as a therapeutic milieu in which the emotional growth of children, parents, and staff occurs.

For the psychiatrist there is practice in how to cooperate with a mental health team. Cooperation with allied fields is not taught in medical school, where the prospective doctor is considered coequal only with researchers.

The psychiatric role becomes clearer in working with a team. Contrary to the common misconception that close interdisciplinary work leads to a blurring of boundaries, the opposite is true: the identity of a discipline sharpens when it collaborates with another discipline.

REFERENCES

1. Bowlby, J., *et al.:* Maternal Care and Mental Health; Deprivation of Maternal Care: A Reassessment of Its Effects. ed. 2. New York, Schocken Books, 1966.
2. Bowlby, J.: Childhood mourning and its implications for psychiatry. Amer. J. Psychiat., *118*:481, 1961.
3. Fagin, C. M.: The Effects of Maternal Attendance During Hospitalization on the Post–Hospital Behavior of Young Children: A Comparative Survey. pp. 61-65. Philadelphia, F. A. Davis, 1966.
4. Robertson, J.: Young Children in Hositals. pp. 20-23. London, Tavistock Publications, 1958.
5. ————: Young Children in Hospitals. p. 14. London, Tavistock Publications, 1958.
6. Bowlby, J., *et al.:* Maternal Care and Mental Health; Deprivation of Maternal Care: A Reassessment of Its Effects. ed. 2. New York, Schocken Books, 1966.
7. Fraiberg, S. H.: The Magic Years. pp. 76-83. New York, C. Scribner's Sons, 1959.

BIBLIOGRAPHY

Bergmann, T., and Freud, A.: Children in the Hospital. New York, International Universities Press, 1965.
Bernstein, N. R., Sanger, S., and Fras, I.: The functions of the child psychiatrist in the management of severely burned children. *In* Chess, S., and Thomas, A. (eds.): Annual Progress in Child Psychiatry and Child Development. New York, Brunner/Mazel, 1970.
Blake, F.: The Child, His Parents and The Nurse. Philadelphia, J. B. Lippincott, 1954.
Blom, G. E.: The reactions of hospitalized children to illness. Pediatrics, *22*:590, 1958.

Bowlby, J.: Child Care and the Growth of Love. ed. 2. Baltimore, Penguin Books, 1965.
————: Attachment and Loss. vol. 1. Attachment. New York, Basic Books, 1969.
Erickson, F.: Nurse specialist for children. Nurs. Outlook, *16*:34, 1968.
Godfrey, A. E.: A study of nursing care designed to assist hospitalized children and their parents in their separation. Nurs. Res., *4*:52, 1955.
Goldfarb, W.: Psychological privation in infancy and subsequent adjustment. Amer. J. Orthopsychiat., *15*:247, 1945.
Gordon, B.: A psychoanalytic contribution to pediatrics. *In* Eissler, R., *et al.:* The Psychoanalytic Study of the Child. vol. 25. New York, International Universities Press, 1970.
Green, M.: Comprehensive pediatrics and the changing role of the pediatrician. *In* Solnit, A. J., and Provence, S. A. (eds.): Modern Perspectives in Child Development. New York, International Universities Press, 1963.
Hamovitch, M. B.: The Parent and the Fatally Ill Child. Los Angeles, Delmar Publishing Co., 1964.
Hirschberg, J. C.: The basic functions of a child psychiatrist in any setting. J. Amer. Acad. Child Psychiat., *5*:360, 1966.
Jessner, L., *et al.:* Emotional implications of tonsillectomy and adenoidectomy on children. *In* Eissler, R., *et al.:* The Psychoanalytic Study of the Child. vol. 7. New York, International Universities Press, 1952.
Levy, D. M.: Psychic traumas of operations in Children. Amer. J. Dis. Child., *69*:7, 1945.
Lickorish, J. R.: The psychometric assessment of the family. *In* Howells, J. G., (ed.): Theory and Practice of Family Psychiatry. New York, Brunner/Mazel, 1971.

Lourie, R. S.: The teaching of child psychiatry in pediatrics. J. Amer. Acad. Child Psychiat., *1*:477, 1962.

McDonald, M.: The psychiatric evaluation of children. J. Amer. Acad. Child Psychiat., *4*:569, 1965.

Murphy, L. B.: Assessment of infants and young children. *In* Chandler, C., *et al.:* Early Child Care: The New Perspectives. New York, Atherton Press, 1968.

Nagera, H.: Children's reactions to death of important objects: a developmental approach. *In* Eissler, R., *et al.* (eds.): The Psychoanalytic Study of the Child. vol. 25. New York, International Universities Press, 1970.

Provence, S. A., and Lipton, R.: Infants in Institutions. New York, International Universities Press, 1962.

Prugh, D. G., *et al.:* A study of the emotional responses of children and families to hospitalization and illness. Amer. J. Orthopsychiat., *23*:70, 1953.

Schaeffer, A. J.: Advantages of mother living in with her hospitalized child. *In* Haller, A., *et al.:* The Hospitalized Child and His Family. Baltimore, Johns Hopkins Press, 1967.

Schulman, J. L.: Management of Emotional Disorders in Pediatric Practice. pp. 109-239. Chicago, Yearbook Medical Publishers, 1967.

Senn, M. J. E., and Solnit, A. J.: Problems in Child Behavior and Development. Chap. 8. Pediatric evaluation. Philadelphia, Lea & Febiger, 1968.

Shirley, H. F.: Pediatric Psychiatry. pp. 642-645. Cambridge, Harvard University Press, 1963.

Shore, M. F. (ed.): Red is the Color of Hurting: Planning for Children in the Hospital. Bethesda, Md., National Institute for Mental Health, 1967.

Silberstein, R. M., *et al.:* Autoerotic head banging; a reflection on the opportunism of infants. J. Amer. Acad. Child Psychiat., *5*:235, 1966.

Solnit, A. J., and Stark, M. H.: Mourning and the birth of a defective child. *In* Eissler, R., *et al.* (eds.): Psychoanalytic Study of the Child. vol. 16, p. 523. New York, International Universities Press, 1961.

Sperling, M.: Asthma in children. An evaluation of concepts and theories. J. Amer. Acad. Child Psychiat., *7*:44, 1968.

Wolf, A. W. M.: Helping Your Child Understand Death. New York, Child Study Association of America Publications, 1958.

Wolf, R. E.: The hospital and the child. *In* Solnit, A. J., and Provence, S. A. (eds.): Modern Perspectives in Child Development. New York, International Universities Press, 1963.

5

Play in the Hospital

IMPORTANCE OF PLAY

Although play and all its functions are not fully understood, existing knowledge indicates that it is crucial for mental health in children. Erikson writes that "to play out is the most natural auto-therapeutic measure childhood affords. Whatever other roles play may have in the child's development . . . the child uses it to make up for defeats, sufferings and frustrations."[1]

Play is a natural phenomenon that leads to learning; it is imaginative, yet is related to reality. Play also fosters and reflects the complexities in the style of emotional development. Through play, the young child expresses his feelings—fantasies, fears and conflicts—in an effort to cope with them, and in so doing he moves toward psychologically more mature behavior.

Every child, healthy or disturbed, is constantly faced with experiences which cause resentments, deprivations and crises. Illness and hospitalization constitute a major stress in early development. They effect a profound change in the child's life style; he faces separation from his parents and from the security of home routines. He also finds himself at the mercy of a hostile environment—a world of unfamiliar sights, sounds and smells, and of strange people who inflict pain. Tensions increase in this anxiety provoking atmosphere, especially when facilities for maintaining normal activity are not available. Play restores, in part, normal aspects of living and prevents further disturbance. Also, it provides the child with the opportunity to reorganize his life; thus, it reduces anxiety and establishes a sense of perspective. When the opportunity for play is not available, destructive and unmanageable behavior is frequently the outcome.

Without suitable communication to enable the child to share his ideas during the actual period of stress, he may find methods that deal with his feelings in a pathological manner. These methods create difficulties in themselves, while the stress may go unrecognized and permanently unresolved.

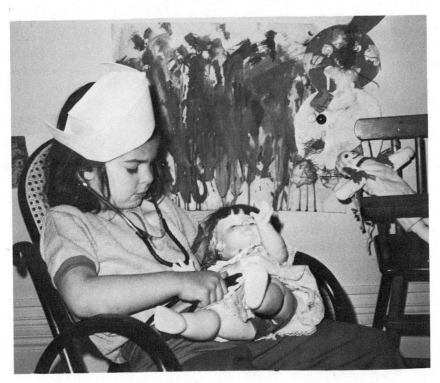

Fig. 5-1. This child casually incorporates new experiences in her play.
(photo by Sirgay Sanger)

Ian was ultimately found to have been preoccupied with the fear that his younger and more charming brother would usurp his toys and family position during his hospital stay. This, unfortunately, he could not articulate. From the moment of his arrival, the staff observed that Ian was a sly, sad 8-year-old who managed to fill his night table with other children's possessions. He was reprimanded for doing so, and he became sadder and withdrawn. The only way he had of telling his problem—acting a caricature of what he feared his brother was doing at home—only brought him more abuse from the environment.

HELPING CHILDREN RECOGNIZE THEIR FEELINGS

Children can be helped to recognize the feelings they are expressing when their moods and words are skillfully reflected back to them.[2] Because of their 24-hour impact, hospital personnel are in an excellent position to help during a stressful period by not allowing feelings to be suppressed.

Jerry was praised by the medical staff as a model patient during an exhaustive "work-up" for diabetes. When a nurse from his unit arrived in the playroom to pick him up for another procedure, she found him putting the finishing touches on a painting and said to him, "This painting must have a story."
Jerry: "Yea, but I can't tell it until I leave. It's a story about my floor—4."
Nurse: "It's a story that can't be told until later?"
Jerry: "Yea."
Nurse: "How come? I won't be scared."
Jerry: "It's about murders. That's all I have to say."
Nurse: "Murders?"

Jerry gave no answer. The nurse sat down looking at the painting.
Jerry said a moment later, "Yea . . ." (in a whisper) ". . . doctors' murders. See here . . ." (pointing to a purple figure) ". . . this means doctors. They're going to get it. I'll show them."
Nurse: "Some pretty awful things must have happened to make you so angry with them."
Jerry: "Yea, lots. They kept hurting me—poking and pinching— and they won't let me eat, and they keep me here. See this?" (pointing to a ceiling light in the painting). "It's not a light. It's really a bomb, and it's going off 2 days after I leave. See this?" (pointing to a red figure). "This means nurses. They're not so bad. Some of them are pretty nice—except that they give needles."

Although he is suffering in silence, Jerry illustrates a child who feels rage toward powerful adults. Children who do not bother the staff may be overlooked. Social conformity is not necessarily an indication of good adjustment. In Jerry's case, closer scrutiny indicated long-standing difficulties with his mother, which he soon acknowledged by complaining of her unwillingness to care for him during this illness. The family required follow-up by social service on a long-term basis.

HELPING CHILDREN COPE WITH A NEW PERCEPTION

Irving could not believe his eyes. He saw 2 body outlines, male and female, in the treatment room of the miniature hospital. He turned to his mother and said accusingly, "You mean to say you don't have a penis?" It was news to this 5-year-old. His mother turned away in disgust saying, "I don't know anything about these things, ask the nurse."

The supportive hospital setting allowed him to pursue this novelty (see Piaget, Chapter 2).

HELPING CHILDREN WHO ARE FEARFUL OF ABANDONMENT

> Cole, age 3, delighted in playing with his own small dollhouse. Casual observation of him during morning care showed his pre-occupation. He knocked on the front door saying repeatedly, "Why won't anyone answer?" Finally, a small female figure from within spoke to him, "This is Amy. Don't you know you don't live here anymore?" His nurse quickly picked up the toy figure and reopened the drama, "This is Amy again, Cole. I bet I fooled you. Sometimes I like to tease. Mamma says you'll be coming home again soon, and that you'll be well again. Then we can have fun. We all miss you." This timely intervention brought a large smile to Cole's face. He played this interchange over and over.

HELPING CHILDREN COMPREHEND THREATENING AND MYSTERIOUS OCCURRENCES IN THE HOSPITAL

> The staff on the unit complimented themselves on their clever-ness in keeping the knowledge of Roger's death from all the other children. His body was taken away in the middle of the night. Both the nurses and doctors reasoned that there was no need to deal with such a delicate problem because no one witnessed the event, and no one asked about Roger. They were chagrined to learn that the children undertook to solve the riddle themselves because the adults were obviously deceitful. Several boys be-tween the ages of 5 and 10 had constructed a coffin out of large building blocks and were playing mortician. Each boy carefully took turns lying in the box, arranging his head in a comfortable elevated position, crossing his arms, and having a sheet gently placed over him.

Even a young child can playfully reenact a new event and become more comfortable.

> Mitzi, 11 months, cried a great deal when a nose culture was taken. After the procedure, her nurse tried to distract her by placing her crib by the window so that she could look out. In this location, the baby was able to reach the supply shelf. She grabbed a handful of applicators and immediately began stuffing them into her doll's nostrils.

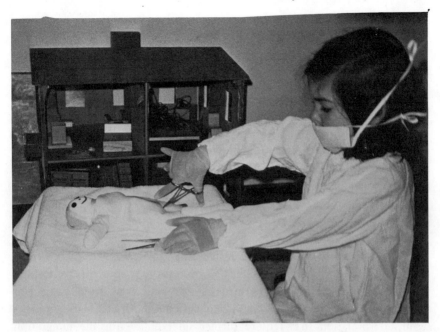

Fig. 5-2. Each child uses supplies in her own way to reenact events that are stressful. (photo by Sirgay Sanger)

HELPING CHILDREN TO CLARIFY DISTORTIONS RECEIVED FROM PARENTS

Maury waited for his mother to leave before calling his nurse. Maury: "Hey, can we do an operation now before my mother gets back? She gets very upset when I operate. You be the nurse and I'll call you up to tell you what I want." (Pretends to call from the nurses' station of the play hospital.) "Hello Miss K., this is Doctor M. I have a young boy here who needs to have a kidney transplant right away."

Miss K: "What is a kidney transplant?"

Maury: "This large green tube like a beanstalk is put into a big hole in the belly."

Miss K.: "That's a new and unusual operation. Sounds like something the gardener uses outside this window. We don't do it on people. Let's talk about the green tube later. Meanwhile what's the patients' name and age?"

Maury: "Oh, you know. It's Maury. He's 5."

Miss K.: "Maury? I know a Maury. There's nothing wrong with his kidneys, doctor. He had a bladder repair (for exstrophy of

the bladder), and he's doing very well now. This boy does not
need more surgery."

Maury: "Are you sure? How come his mother said, 'The next
thing I hear, you'll be needing a kidney transplant'?"

Maury had been exposed to his mother's alarming and confusing words.
His hospitalization for long periods allowed the staff to form relationships
that served to clarify his illness and buffer him against the confusion at
home. He went on to inform his mother and siblings of the true nature of
his hospitalization, insisting she hear the facts. When she doubted them, he
arranged a conference between her and a house officer.

DIAGNOSTIC USE OF PLAY

Play is an important diagnostic instrument. It increases our knowledge
of the child's mental life—of his deeper reactions to events. In the hospital
setting, play reflects the child's meaning of being away from home and
the effects of medical routines and personnel on him. It can highlight areas
of misinterpretation that require further intervention for the integration
of experiences.

WHAT CAN BE LEARNED FROM CHANCE OBSERVATION

Following circumcision, Howie, age 5, was asked by a recreation worker what kind of operation he was doing on his doll. He
replied that he was cutting off the penis so that he could give it a
new one.

Four-year-old Lew was serenely stringing beads. Occasionally,
he looked about the playroom; then, suddenly he dashed into an
adjoining room in which the play hospital was located. Working
against time, he toppled the furniture, threw doctor and nurse dolls
into the waste basket, and destroyed the most fragile equipment.
Within 10 seconds, he returned to his seat and resumed work,
quite unaware that he had been observed.

Lucy, age 6, was found playing doctor and saying to her doll,
"If you don't hold still, I'm going to stick you 10 times."

A staff, alert to the importance of play, can make observations such as
with Howie, Lew, and Lucy several times a day. These observations may
require immediate intervention, but usually they can be postponed until
they are discussed at the mental health team conferences.

WHAT CAN BE LEARNED WITH MORE DELIBERATE ATTENTION TO THE SUBTLETIES OF PLAY

Closer observation of play indicates a child's developmental level (see Chapter 2). Other characteristics the staff will learn to look for are *regression in the presence of frustration* and *reversibility of the regression.* For example, when told he could not leave his bed, Arnold, age 5 began to throw his food at the informant. When told what the reason was for being in bed, he became cooperative and curious about the x-ray he would be having. Another child may not have stopped so readily. The regressive behavior—food throwing—was short-lived. He resumed socially acceptable behavior promptly. Play can reveal many of these regressive and reversible reactions.

However, a reaction that appears ominous in overt behavior may show a more benign perspective in play. For example, 9-year-old Ben was told on Monday he would have a bone marrow biopsy on Wednesday. The procedure was postponed twice. By the end of the week he was overheard whispering to his roommate that the staff were not to be trusted and were trying to keep the children guessing as to their future. In the playroom, he played a cowboy who was very angry at being cheated by the gambler. It emerged that Ben saw the doctor as a person who was untrustworthy. His seemingly pathological suspiciousness disappeared when the delay was discussed.

The following examples illustrate children's views of the many events that occur while they are hospitalized and how first appearances can be deceptive.

Craig, age 7, required elaborate preparation before heart surgery because he also had a blood disorder. The postoperative period was amazingly uneventful except that the child developed an intense fear of having his finger pricked daily for blood work. His reactions were discussed with the lab technician who was told how to play with the child. She asked him why his friend across the hall was afraid of needles; Craig did not know. The next time blood was drawn, the technician asked John, the friend, to visit at Craig's bedside where John pretended to use a syringe on a stuffed kangaroo. Seeing this, Craig said to him, "You can't take blood that way. Don't you know he has to have a transfusion after each test? Losing too much blood can kill you!"

Cyrena, age 12, asked her nurse to use miniature equipment to prepare her for open heart surgery. She asked many questions but gave no clue to her preoccupation until the end of the session. The child played beautifully. She had the parents sweetly waving good-bye and a nurse accompanying the tiny patient to the treatment room. She revealed that she had a detailed knowledge of the heart. The nurse was startled when, from the doorway, she saw Cyrena pull a sheet over the doll's head and say, "That's it, she's dead!"

HOW THE CHILDREN VIEW THE STAFF

Because of his lengthy hospitalization, the staff made arrangements for Peter, age 9, to go down to the pediatric lobby in order to visit his younger siblings. Just before one visit, he prepared an album about his hospital experiences so that his brothers and sisters would know what he was experiencing. His favorite drawing showed a patient in the process of a kidney biopsy. He used it as a visual aid to illustrate his story to the family. "Well," he said, "some people think they know it all. I tried to tell the doctor that I couldn't hold still in that position but she said I was being silly. I said it was cold; she said it was just right. O.K. for her, she was dressed up to her ears in a gown, cap and mask and there I was cold and practically naked. She said I wouldn't feel any pain; I said I did. She said she'd get it (the specimen) the first time; I know she didn't. So who the hell would know better?"

The mental health team was alerted by the child's accurate perception of a serious problem in a staff member. This doctor was known for her "no nonsense" approach to procedures. Efforts were made to show the doctor how the child's use of the words cold and naked was symbolic of the effect of her perfunctory approach. She did not agree with this criticism and said that she had an excellent rapport with Peter.

Matt, age 8, who had leukemia, was encouraged to paint pictures of his hospital experiences. After a period of isolation (when his resistance to infection was low), he produced a series of paintings that he distributed to members of the pediatric staff. The repetitive theme of the paintings showed a very small boy shackled to a large treatment table. Two doctors stood by, making attacking gestures with syringes and needles larger than the boy's body.

A more vivid demonstration of the way play reveals children's views of the staff was exemplified by large posters. These posters were thinly veiled, hostile, manifestations of the children's feelings.

The older boys on the ward mischievously tacked up signs expressing their feelings regarding treatments and the nursing staff. Kevin, age 10, wrote, "Wanted. Nurse _____ who is unfair to children. Forty dollars reward." Then he drew her likeness in profile and full face.

Edward, age 12, posted a sign on his door to keep intruders away. It said, "Beware of Mad Dogs. Will get anyone with needles."

This approach is the closest many children get toward expressing their anger and fear; however, it does not go far enough. The staff can take advantage of these clues to channel covert aspects of hostility into workable verbalization.

A useful technique for this is to have relevant staff apologize for painful treatments. An apology can have various reactions. One effect is to encourage brashness with those children who are preoccupied with power struggles in their relationships. The child sees this kind of apology as weakness in the staff; thus, the child thinks he can be rude. The other effect is to offer the child an example of an adult who compromises. If the child is looking for a grown-up with whom to identify, he will suppress further hostility in order to emulate this model. Therefore, if alerted to the reactions, an adult who apologizes can assay whether the patient is early phallic (competitive) or late phallic (concerned with gender identification). (See Chapter 2.)

Daryl, age 5, was recovering from circumcision. He painted a picture and told the story of a bomber that passed over his house and destroyed everything in sight. He said that it took 3 days for the sun to come out again. On that third day, he had received sympathy and an apology for his condition.

The circumcision had defeated Daryl's competitive spirit and caused him to feel vanquished. Only after Daryl had checked out the environment did he feel strong enough to reveal his sunshine.

Manny, age 8, was so nasty that he alienated most of the staff with his laughing and provocative actions. After the incision and drainage of a large abscess, he painted a picture of Batman and Robin in a Batmobile, rushing to a cave entrance in order to get away from black raindrops. First, Manny wanted to show this painting to his favorite nurse, but then he decided not to. He said his roommate would understand his picture better and painted another one in its place. This picture was a large flower pot with several bright flowers and small green raindrops surrounding them. When the nurse asked him for a story he said, "What's the matter with you? Can't you see? It's a pot with dirt. These are flowers and the rain is making things come up good."

Manny shows the progression from early phallic preoccupation—picturing Batman hiding in a cave to avoid danger—to the boldly visible late phallic exuberance—picturing large bright flowers in a pot. This mirrored a change in staff attitudes from punitive, repressive control toward more supportive, individualized care. The evidence obtained from the paintings helped the mental health team to continue in the latter direction against strong pressures to be vindictive.

DETERMINING THE BASIS OF A PROBLEM

While Dossie was recovering from surgery for the reimplantation of a ureter, her mother complained that the child was chronically constipated. She asked the pediatrician to investigate the problem during Dossie's hospitalization. Observations made by the nurses indicated that a severe conflict existed between the mother and the 3-year-old. As a result, diagnostic medical studies were postponed until more information could be obtained. It was characteristic of this mother to create situations that were frustrating for the child. When visiting her daughter she spent much time playing with the small babies on the unit. She could not understand Dossie's jealousy and rage because none of this behavior had occurred at home; Dossie had an 8-month-old sibling.

Further observations were made in the play hospital where Dossie collected several infant dolls from the nursery and deposited them on the operating table, in the toilet bowl and in waste baskets. As Dossie continued, the nurse remarked that she played with babies a great deal. "Yes," she said, "I like babies—except when they cry or when they are held." This was the natural opening for the nurse to discuss with Dossie her negative feelings toward her sibling, and to encourage her to demand her mother's attention. Within seconds Dossie ran out to the bathroom and had a normal bowel movement. She returned quite relaxed and announced that she wanted to play again. This time she concentrated on doctor dolls and placed several doctors around the bed of a little girl doll. When she was asked what the doctors were doing she said, "They're scaring the BM out."

Additional sessions produced similar material followed by trips to the bathroom. Consequently, Dossie no longer needed diagnostic testing. Instead, her mother was referred to a social worker who arranged counseling to ameliorate her frustration. Dossie increasingly used words to signify her anger; thus, she limited the attack, in the form of constipation, that she had formerly used against her mother. This case illustrates a deep oppositional struggle between a parent and child (see Chapter 2).

EVALUATING THE EFFECTIVENESS OF PREOPERATIVE TEACHING

Although Abe, age 5, received thorough preparation for heart surgery, his play later revealed that his preoccupations were not touched upon. He explained to his father who was watching him manipulate his teaching doll, "This kid has 3 holes in his heart, and he's a dead duck."

Cory, age 4, had been carefully prepared for a tonsillectomy. It was clear that he did not retain the information for long. In playing with his teaching doll postoperatively, he kept mentioning, "Don't take off the boy's pants." Hearing this, his nurse remembered that Cory had objected violently to being completely undressed, except for a johnny shirt, prior to surgery. This indicated that additional teaching was required, and that the arbitrary policy of removing all undergarments before any operation only reinforced the child's fantasy of having other parts of the body operated upon. The policy was immediately changed with the cooperation of the operating room staff.

The Usefulness of Play in Groups

"In group play . . . children assign to themselves roles which are an expression or an extension of their basic problems. In such roles, one either plays out the awareness of what he is, or a hopeful phantasy of what he would like to be. . . . In a group such phantasies are reinforced and find easy and natural means of coming through in a variety of play forms and activity channels.[3]

The sight of others pretending and freely showing their concerns, serves as a stimulus and gives to the less playful child, permission to do the same thing. This child finds companionship and some sympathy in his difficulty;

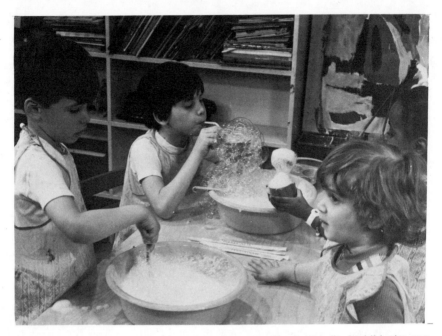

Fig. 5-3. Group play consists of both imaginary and real stimuli. A child who can only allow one or the other is quickly revealed. (photo taken from the film "Play in the Hospital," Play School Association, Campus Films)

however, he is not allowed to feel sorry for himself. Group sessions also inform children that others have similar feelings.

A group often takes up issues that would not be seen in individual play, such as sibling competition for the adult's attention.

If the group is sufficiently cohesive it establishes values that impose certain restraints on unsociable behavior. Seeing how others cope, especially if they are younger and sicker, is an impressive learning experience. Group interaction may speed the possibility of positive affectionate role playing; on the other hand, it can be frightening to see how other children fail to cope. Any upset could be profitably used by recreation workers and other staff in later conversation and play with an individual child.

Group play consists of both imaginary and real stimuli. The child who can only allow one stimulus or the other is quickly revealed. The highly imaginative child may be out of touch with others. The excessively practical child may be dully anchored to concrete events. The well-adjusted child needs and allows both stimuli.

TECHNIQUES OF PLAY

Initially it is important to get clues to a child's more obvious preoccupations. Some knowledge of his real circumstances makes possible individualized play approaches. Chance remarks picked up from the staff are helpful; e.g., "After all Josh has been through, his only objection is to the daily finger pricks," or "How odd for Mrs. D. to go on vacation while her child is hospitalized," or "Every time I pass Maury he tries to get me to play doctor games with him."

There are general rules that can be applied whenever effective play is to be initiated:

- Reflect only what the child expresses.
- Supply materials which stimulate play.
- Allow enough time without interruption.
- Permit a child to play at his own pace.
- Determine when it is appropriate to go beyond the child's expression.
- Play for the child who cannot play for himself.
- Allow direct play for the emotionally strong child. Be familiar with some artistic material as a medium of expression.
- Have a knowledge of child growth and development because it guides the professional in clinical judgement.

REFLECTING ONLY WHAT THE CHILD EXPRESSES

It is axiomatic that the creation of a play situation is based on a secure atmosphere. Unfamiliar words and ideas threaten a child, leading to the inhibition of his spontaneity.

> While Connie was hospitalized, her mother took the opportunity to go on vacation; however, this was never directly mentioned by the child. Play with cutouts of Orphan Annie and Sandy revealed her true feelings. In one episode, Orphan Annie, after having abandoned Sandy, her canine friend, returned from the North Pole and picked him up at the kennel. Sandy whimpered and scolded her mercilessly. The nurse asked Connie what the dog was saying. Connie insisted that he had hated being left. The nurse sympathized with Sandy by saying that it wasn't pleasant being left behind with no one to play with and being all alone in a little box with only strangers around; he had a right to be angry. However, Connie did not agree saying, "But he's only a dog."

It was obvious that Connie was not ready to admit her anger; therefore the nurse did not go beyond the child's expression. The nurse had confidence that eventually Connie would be candid and would admit her anger as she felt more secure in her relationship with the nurse.

SUPPLYING MATERIALS FOR PLAY

Any toys and materials that children use are immediately invested with imaginative qualities. Then these concrete objects become suitable vehicles for carrying out structured fantasies about the child's most current preoccupations. The clarity of the themes will vary depending on the degree of anxiety generated. Too much anxiety and the child will conceal the problem, try to change the subject, or stop playing altogether. Also these actions are efforts by the child to cope with the same anxiety-provoking theme, though the external manifestation appears to be different; therefore, the staff should not be misled. A child will remain preoccupied with the main challenge to his safety until it is met in some way.

> In his play, Teddy continually wanted objects to fall off, such as the smokestacks on ships and the wings of planes. This obvious castration fear appeared to vanish when he stopped his aeronautical drawings and rushed to the window to exclaim about the missing screens. However, his first observation of missing screens was merely a continuation of the same fear.

The child who is in the grip of a specific conflict will return to it constantly. Nonetheless, he will use many disguises until he finds one that gives him sufficient distance to cope with the danger in order to achieve a happier solution.

For Teddy, the use of toy planes, boats and other transportation toys resulted in monotonous play. Even the windows of the elegant playhouse seemed unproductive of discussion. Only when he asked for another tongue depressor did he become animated—filling in an empty space in a wooden bridge he was building with tongue depressors. It was the closest he could comfortably get to castration anxiety. From this point he was able to gradually approach this anxiety by way of fallen screens, fallen wings, and finally fallen "things."

This case shows that the play materials did not fit this boy's needs until he was allowed to choose his own media.

> Veronica set up a bed, croupette and a bedside stand. She brought in a medicine dropper and cup on a tray placing them on

the table. As she opened the croupette she said to the two dolls, "I'm putting you two in bed together. You'll be happier that way. Now I have to put this flap back so I can get to you two with triple measles. Now, now, don't cry, this medicine is good for you. It tastes just like cookies and you know you only get good cookies in the hospital, not like at home."

This play sequence was made possible by the use of materials attractive and relevant to the child's experiences in the hospital. Real cookies were made available for play. Eventually, the staff realized that the cookies symbolized "starving" for affection at home. On interview with the parents, the social worker confirmed this play diagnosis.

ALLOWING THE CHILD TO PROCEED AT HIS OWN PACE

A child cannot be rushed into approaching frightening ideas and changes in body functions.

> Five-year-old Millie completely rejected preoperative teaching for an ileo-conduit. She pulled off the play equipment—I.V., drainage bags, and dressings from the teaching doll and appeared to ignore any mention of impending surgery. Postoperatively, she was withdrawn, refused to look at the operative site, and denied that she knew what had happened to her. An indirect approach was used with her because direct teaching upset her greatly. A box of equipment—tubes, small bottles, dressings, and pediatric urine collectors (PUC to represent "ostomy" bags)—was left at her bedside without comment. On the next day, the nurse observed that the PUC was attached to the doll's head. She made no mention of this. On the following day the PUC moved to the right arm, and on the third day it moved to the chest. On the fourth day, it appeared on the abdomen. Concomitantly, Millie was able to look at the operative site and to talk about the procedure directly.

GOING BEYOND THE CHILD'S EXPRESSIONS

In selected cases it is permissible to say things in play beyond what the child is expressing superficially. This gives the anxious child a chance to see that someone else can talk about a frightening topic and continue to be friendly. It gives security to find a companion for sharing fears.

> Patsy, age 8, suffered traumatic injury to one eye, followed by a severe infection that led to blindness in that eye. She was encouraged to reenact the treatments she experienced on her

patient doll—injections, I.V.'s, warm soaks, and changing of dressings—as a way of stimulating discussion about the accident and
its consequences. In playing the part of the doll, her nurse
expressed concern for the outcome of treatment—of how her sight
would be affected. However, Patsy denied the loss of her vision
and told the nurse that she could see through the bandage.

Because of impending surgery, a time limitation made it necessary to accelerate her play; so that she could face what she was
trying to avoid. It was important for her nurse to let Patsy know
that there was no sight through the bandage, and that the staff
was concerned about her vision. She needed to realize that the
doctors could not promise a good treatment result though they
hoped for the best in treating the infection.

On the day before surgery, the idea of enucleation had to be
broached with her. The pediatrician and mental health nurse first
discussed this with the mother, who asked the staff to tell Patsy
about the enucleation. These parents were thought to use deception when under stress; therefore, the doctor and nurse who knew
Patsy best decided on a joint approach.

The doctor was to take the strong position about the reality;
the nurse was to offer comfort and solace. Both doctor and nurse
respected this youngster's dignity and bravery in the face of a
mutilating experience.

Nurse: "You've probably been thinking a lot about the conversations we've had all week and you might have some worries about
what we've said."

Patsy nods her head.

Nurse: "What do you do when unpleasant thoughts come to your
head."

Patsy: "I put them under the pillow."

Nurse: "And they don't go away, do they?"

Patsy nods.

Nurse: "That's why we have to talk about them. Sometimes
they're easier to take when you share them with someone else. Do
you have an idea why the doctor is with me today?"

Patsy shakes her head as if she knows but doesn't want to hear.

Doctor: "Patsy, we've done everything possible to clear up the
infection but we couldn't do enough. You know we've been worried about your eye and we have just come to the conclusion that
there is nothing more we can do to make it better and to save the
sight in your eye."

Nurse: (observing tears in Patsy's eye) "It makes you feel like crying, doesn't it?"
Patsy begins to cry.
Nurse: "You've got a lot to cry about. It's okay to cry."
The nurse stayed with Patsy until her mother arrived to offer comfort.

PLAYING FOR A CHILD WHO CANNOT PLAY FOR HIMSELF

Liam, age 2½, was extensively burned over his entire body; as a result, he was completely immobilized. All he had for coping with the problem was an extraordinary capacity for speech and an inquisitive mind.

The staff in the Intensive Care Unit requested the help of the nursing mental health consultant for the emotional aspects of his care. Liam was calling himself a bad boy, and refusing to talk about the accident.

Play with this child was a challenge—complicated by the fact that he was unable to participate directly, and because of the need for aseptic techniques such as wearing cap, gown, mask and gloves. Initially, stories were used as a way of establishing rapport. It was hoped that later he might be able to explore the theme of blame and guilt.

A modified version of the 3 bears in which the facts of Liam's own hospitalization were inserted served the purpose: Goldilocks, a very curious child, investigated the bears' home, trying out everything including Baby Bear's own chair. Because she was too large for it, she broke the chair, but fixed it so it did not look broken. On Baby Bear's return, he sat on his favorite chair, fell, and hurt himself very badly. He did not know that it was broken; it was not his fault. Momma and Poppa Bear rushed him to the hospital in Police Chief Bear's private car so that the doctors and nurses could care for him.

Once Baby Bear got to the hospital, he needed to have the bumps and sores on his body cleaned. He also needed medicines and bandages to make him feel better, and he needed extra food and medicines through a little tube in his arm. (This was shown to a little teddy bear because he was curious and wanted to know what was going on.)

As this story was told treatment was demonstrated and explained to Liam on a doll and with play equipment sterilized for this occasion. Because he could not use his body except for his eyes and mouth, he watched while the figure was animated for him.

The bear story continued: Once Baby Bear was treated at the hospital, a doctor asked him how he had gotten hurt. Baby Bear said that he was a bad bear, but of course, that was not true. If he had known that the chair was broken, he would not have sat in it, and if Momma and Poppa Bear knew that he was in danger they would have come to help him. The accident was not their fault either.

After listening to the story attentively, Liam asked, "How did I get on the stove?"

The question was turned back to him, "I don't know. How did you get up there?"

He was then willing to tell, "I climbed up there and got burned." He was assured that it was not his fault; he did not know that the stove was hot. He just wanted to find out what it was all about because he was a curious boy—and usually curiosity is a safe thing to follow. Liam smiled and asked to have his Snoopy dog brought near. This request indicated that he was once more interested in his transitional object as he had been before the accident.

On one occasion Liam said that his father looked like a baker in his isolation gown and cap. He was asked what bakers did, and he responded that they made cookies. Liam was told that he too could make cookies in the playroom when he was better. He declined saying, "I can't because I got burned." He was told that there were safe ways to make cookies without getting burned again.

There are a number of children who because of their illness or physical defects cannot use their bodies in play. For these children the staff must assume the dialectic process. In this way, the child will select with his eyes or with words what issues he is grappling with. In Liam's case his intense curiosity was used to re-experience his accident and to support and recommence his developmental growth. He became quite happy and in touch with his family and visitors despite his immobility.

Even though he died several weeks later, the staff and family felt that the efforts were worthwhile because Liam was his usual delightful self, right to the end.

PLAYING WITH AN EMOTIONALLY STRONG CHILD

Some children can tolerate thematic expression that is quite close to a painful reality.

Several boys wearing leg bags for urinary drainage were gathered around the water trough. Will picked up a large syringe and accidentally discovered that it had three streams of water. He was delighted, and he showed the syringe to the other boys repeatedly. Will, hospitalized for repair of hypospadias, had that number of streams when he voided. In this case, no complex intervention in play was required. Instead the large syringe was given to Will for the next few days. He tried a variety of colored liquids in his experiments. When the doctors came to his bed on rounds, he played a practical joke by suddenly showing his sprayer syringe in all its glory.

Hanna stood before the mirror in the playroom and put on a long dress and floppy hat. She then packed a suitcase and took Eileen, a younger child with her. Both girls sat on a bench in front of the elevator. Hanna explained that she waiting for a bus to take her and the little girl home. A recreation worker talked to Hanna about her reasonable wish to go home. It was a great relief for her to hear from an adult that home was a place everyone wanted to be.

USING ART MATERIALS

Art materials are particularly suitable for expressing internal concerns.[4] The child must be free to work on his own without direction from adults and without comment on the artistic merit of the production. Each child uses supplies in his own way. Adults need to be completely non-judgmental and to discard preconceived notions on the nature of art. Painting should be treated as symbolic of the child's thoughts, not as an entity in itself. Asking simple questions after the work is completed draws out the youngster's story. With older children it is more productive to talk about the theme that the painting illustrates.

Among 10-year-old Beckie's paintings before surgery for revision of a cleft lip repair, were scenes in which 2 trees were at opposite ends of the paper. The significance of these productions became clear when she resumed her artwork postoperatively. In her first drawing she united the branch of one tree with the other—linking them with an arc similar to the instrument used on her lip to prevent tension on the suture line.

Before surgery, Pearl, age 8, painted a picture of Egypt with pyramids and palms. She explained that she was studying this in school. On the day after surgery for cleft lip repair, she painted a mess of blacks and reds. Two days later she began to reorganize and started again on Egyptian themes. Thus, as long as she could think of the possibility of a complete repair of the anomaly she thought of Egypt—which symbolized to her a beautiful place. The horrible blacks and reds without definition, represented her view of the inside of her mouth.

At a mental health team conference, Pearl's paintings were discussed and psychotherapy was recommended. It appeared as if she would never be satisfied with the surgical result; she had to learn that even with an excellent repair, she would not obtain the exotic, perfect atmosphere of the Egypt that was pictured in her mind. In addition, an effort would have to be made to reconcile the disgust she felt (the mess of black and red) toward the preoperative oral cavity.

Lil, age 11, previously had numerous surgical procedures for a congenital deformity of the leg. On her second postoperative day, she drew a picture of a leg in a cast and a hand with a wedding band close to it. She asked the recreational worker after handing her the picture, "Are you married, Miss W.?"

Miss W. pointed to the picture and said, "Here's someone who is married. Could you tell me about her?"

Lil said the figure in the drawing had found somebody nice and cute, and had married him. She said, "Do you think I'll get married? My cousin didn't get married because her boyfriend had very little hair."

Miss W. asked, "Do you think your leg would make someone change his mind about marrying you?" Lil was thoughtful, but did not reply so Miss W. went on, "I don't know what happened with your cousin, but usually people get married because they have deep feelings for one another, not because of the kind of hair or shape of the leg." (Lil showed a cultural precosity in that at age 11 she had an adolescent's concern about her future marital role.)

It took more than a week to convey this message. After a while her drawings were of entire figures rather than isolated parts of the body.

HOW TO PLAY WHEN THERE ARE NO CLUES ABOUT A CHILD'S PREOPERATIVE CONCERNS

When little is known about a child's inner anxieties, effective play should be related to the chronological level of the child (see Chapter 2). Before age 5, the concerns commonly held by children are abandonment, pain and mutilation, invasion of body orifices, and loss of control over their usual routines. Stories about these themes could be about people who shut their eyes, children who cover their ears, children who are left at doorsteps, or things that are missing or change their appearance.

Themes of mastery start early and continue throughout childhood; for example, pleasure in newness of function and knowledge. These can be expressed in stories about exploring big houses and the hospital, meeting strangers who turn out to be nice, jumping into water and finding it good, and trying new foods and finding them delicious.

For 5- to 10-year-olds, play can be initiated with the following themes: making things that last, acquiring a skill that is better than others', pleasing adults other than parents, being ashamed or losing face, carrying out the usual patterns of living with friends, sports, hobbies and role model activities in the hospital. Other themes might occur in stories that tell of triumph over danger.

Eleven- to 16-year-olds usually dread returning to a dependent position with illness, regard their peer group as the final word on social success, and worry about their occupational choice.

Some commercially available books present, in an attractive way, 1 or 2 developmental tasks. These are depicted by characters or animals with whom the child can identify—neither too close nor too distant from the challenge the child faces. The chief protagonist is sufficiently recognizable to capture the imagination.

The following books are listed according to age. They have held up clinically for hundreds of readings.

TWO-AND-A-HALF TO FOUR YEARS

Wezel, P.: The Good Bird. New York, Harper & Row, 1964. (A fish, all alone, is befriended by a bird and they stay together all night. Told without words.)

Eastman, P.: Are You My Mother?. New York, Random House, 1960. (A bird hatches while his mother has gone to find him a worm; he misses the mother and goes on a long walk to find her. A happy reunion ensues.)

Piper, W.: The Little Engine That Could. New York, Platt, 1954. (An engine almost gives up but finally climbs over a mountain to deliver its toys.)

Mayer, M.: There's a Nightmare In My Closet. New York, Dial Press, 1968. (A boy's premonition of a moster in his closet comes true; however, the monster is more afraid than the boy. The child manages very well in the end.)

Bemelmans, L.: Madeline. New York, Simon and Shuster, 1939. (A girl has an operation, and her friends envy her scar. At first the teacher is hysterical, but then she calms down.)

Cameron, P.: I Can't, Said The Ant. New York, Coward-McCann, 1961. (A broken teapot and spout get mended with great effort and rhyme.)

Sendak, M.: Where The Wild Things Are. New York, Harper & Row, 1963. (A boy who is punished by his mother revels in his badness and returns to a warm supper.)

De Regniers, B. S.: How Joe The Bear and Sam The Mouse Got Together. New York, Parents' Magazine Press, 1965. (Very dissimilar animals find after much negotiation that they both like ice cream.)

THREE TO SEVEN YEARS

Hoban, R.: Bedtime for Frances. New York, Harper & Row, 1960. (A bear has night fears but eventually gets to sleep.)

Minarek, E. H.: Little Bear's Friend. New York, Harper & Row, 1960. (One of the 4 vignettes concerns a doll whose arm needs repair.)

Skorpen, L. M.: That Mean Man. New York, Harper & Row, 1968. (An unsavory character gets his comeuppance, but not before he tries a lot of things that children are told not to do.)

Alexander, M.: We Never Get To Do Anything. New York, Dial Press, 1970. (A boy finds a way to enjoy himself despite the rules.)

Brown, J.: Flat Stanley. New York, Harper & Row, 1964. (A boy makes the best of an accident.)

SIX TO TEN YEARS

Weber, A.: Elizabeth Gets Well. New York, T. Y. Crowell, 1970. (A girl has surgery after which she gets well.)

White, E. B.: Charlotte's Web. New York, Harper & Row, 1952. (Life, death, love, and hard work as illustrated by the relationship between the spider and a pig.)

White, E. B.: The Trumpet of the Swan. New York, Harper & Row, 1970. (How a very human swan overcomes a terrible defect to lead a normal, even exemplary life.)

MASTERY THROUGH PLAY

In the process of growth and development, early egocentricity alters continuously in the direction of sociability. Concomitantly there is a diminution of magical ideas of self-importance as arduously gained skills become the basis for a sense of real importance. For many children, this process is an injury to the self-esteem because they are reminded of their small size, awkwardness and needs for help in growing up. For them hospitalization will reinforce a sense of impotence and helplessness.

These feelings may be expressed and at times surmounted, by playing out stories of powerful and lowly characters. Bible stories (Samson) and some of Aesop's fables contain many passive to active plots. The child will attempt to master situations in which he is a helpless victim by turning passive experiences into active ones.[5] This kind of play should be encouraged.

It is important to ensure the survival of puppets, dolls, or animals that the child treats cruelly or murderously because in power reversal the player may go too far. Children feel secure when they are stopped from excessive destruction of equipment; however when they are engaged in violent non-destructive acts, the play should be allowed to continue, and words should be used as a moderating force. This action is permissible as children learn, in this way, to gradually modulate aggression toward saying instead of doing. Furthermore, only a severely disturbed child would fail to differentiate the animate from the inanimate, and use the violent play against people.

> Several boys were playing after transfusion clinic. Together they started to put several I.V.'s into a large toy bear's body. Before long they were violently attacking the bear, urging each other on.

> Grant underwent a kidney transplant at age 7. His hospitalization was particularly long and complicated. Of all the procedures he required, injections were the hardest for him to bear. There was much play with needles as a way of dealing with the difficulty. This soon led to his building the "Grant Animal Clinic." Each stuffed animal he acquired—snake, tiger, skunk, and dog—became

the new patient whose ailments required extensive treatment with injections. Doctor Grant possessed amazing powers to cure, and before long, had an extensive practice requiring the services of a nurse whom he ordered about. "Make an appointment for him in 3 months; that treatment really did the job." His nurse in turn, complimented him on being able to save even the sickest victims.

Dan, age 5, and others were playing doctors rounds. They surrounded a nurse in the playroom and proceeded to examine her with stethoscopes and tongue depressors. David, 7, said, "I think this patient has to stay in bed for 10 days and we'll give her more medicine."

Everyone agreed except Dan. He said, "Three days. I'm chief here and what I say goes. I've been on rounds before."

Elsie frequently placed her dolls on a stretcher and practiced taking them back and forth from her room to the corridor leading to the operating room. For this 5-year-old, going to the operating room was a familiar trip because she required repeated skin grafting. On one occasion just prior to surgery, she asked her nurse to take her and the dolls for a ride on the stretcher in the same area. She appeared to gain strength from the practice sessions by building up a tolerance for the anxiety the operations provoked.

Edward, age 8, was distressed to learn about heart surgery and to see the miniature teaching equipment. "I don't know how I am going to stand it," he said. And then as an afterthought, "I know what I'll do. I'll ask my father to make toys like this for me."

ORGANIZED PLAY PROGRAMS

Recreation Staff

Therapeutic play programs[6,7,8] are the achievement of full-time professional recreational workers. Extensive education in child development as well as clinical experience with both well and sick children are the basic qualifications. Judgments need to be made continuously on children's coping ability under stress. Thus professonals require a variety of techniques and skills for evaluating and managing behavioral problems in a hospital setting. Preparation is essential for perceiving what a child is thinking and feeling and for answering a child's needs as they emerge in play.

Recreational workers in their non-medical roles are readily accepted by children as supportive adults. They, too, facilitate the expression of fears and anxiety and hasten the process of adaptation.

For most children, to sit down with an adult and to talk on a meaningful level about imaginative issues, is a unique experience. The closeness that a child feels opens up vistas for warmth and acceptance by a powerful larger person that can only lead to increasing optimism about growing up.

Assistants in Play

Volunteers and students of all disciplines are valuable assistants to full-time workers in direct proportion to the amount of orientation and supervision they receive. However, their effectiveness is often limited by the lack of constant staff support. This is made difficult by the fact that most of these people are part-time workers. Nevertheless, with their participation, it is often possible to expand a program by supplying extensive support and companionship for children during treatments, prolonged separation from parents, periods of isolation, and serious illness that prevents attendance in the playroom.

Pediatrics patients can deal with the traumas of hospitalization most effectively in a play area designed specifically for this purpose. Neutral, familiar, and unlike the general hospital territory, the playroom is geared to helping the process of mastery. Here also, children interact with each other and are given free reign to manipulate the environment to the extent their illnesses permit. Given the opportunity, children will seek solutions to situations that perplex them and find suitable outlets for the fear and anger generated by disruptive experiences.

The interaction of recreation, nursing and medical staffs allows for a continuous exchange of information covering the child's 24-hour activities. This contact leads to a continuity of approach and management. Participation of medical personnel in the play program may be reassuring to children because it implies that play is valued and enjoyed by staff who may not have the time to be regularly present in the play area. The children need to know that doctors and nurses are not always associated with pain.

> Debbie, age 12, observed a nurse surrounded by several children, each carrying out different types of needle play. She looked puzzled and finally asked, "What do you do, do you give needles?" Nurse: "Sometimes I do, but I'd rather teach children how to do it so they won't be so frightened."

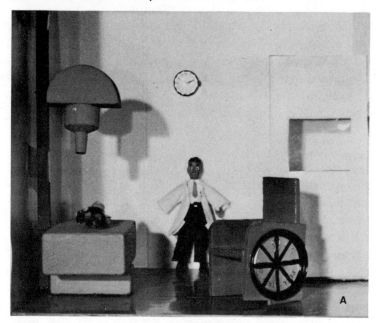

A. X-ray room

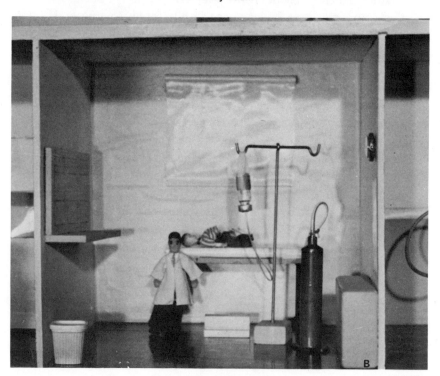

B. Treatment room

Figs. 5-4 A-E. The miniature hospital stimulates imaginative play where intensive feelings are given expression. (photos by Steve Campus)

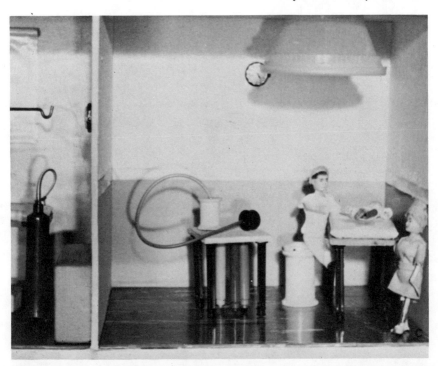

C. Anesthesia room

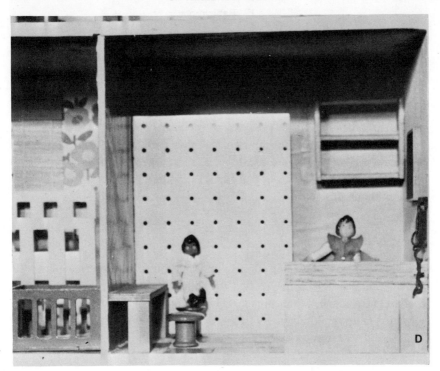

D. Nurses' station

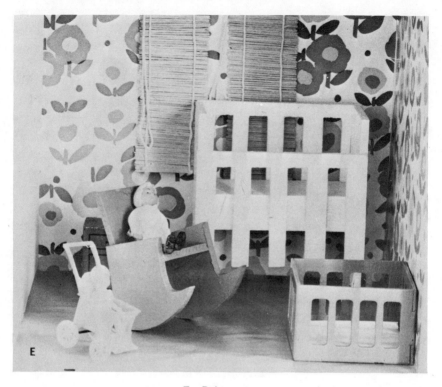

E. Baby room

Debbie: "Well then are you a nurse or are you . . ." (unable to finish question).
Nurse: "Or what, Debbie?"
Debbie: "A child helper?"

On the other hand, the presence of medical personnel in the play area may be threatening if the children feel that their arrival indicates that a treatment will occur on the premises. Children must be able to regard the playrooms (as well as their bedrooms) as safety zones where they may relax without this fear.

Play Materials

The organized play area affords optimal conditions for free play. "In general, play activities are chosen that allow for a variety of approaches, that are unstructured, that can be used by a wide age range, by both boys and girls, by many children at the same time. It is also important to choose those which will stimulate and challenge but which do not impose arbitrary demands of completion in a given form."[9]

Pounding boards, play dough made by children, water play, and painting are excellent for diversion, entertainment and expression of feelings. In addition, the professional knows how to use these activities to create stories and themes when children choose not to use puppets. Play in which children have available miniature beds, stretchers, and wheelchairs stimulate realistic role taking. Blocks, dolls, doll house, and kitchen corner are ideal for preschoolers. Group play is stimulated by supplying several items of a kind and arranging equipment in clusters. The play staff can encourage play around episodes and fears which are significant. The hospital corner with real and toy equipment (dolls representing all personnel of the pediatric department, patient dolls, nurses' caps, stethoscopes, doctor bag containing syringes, alcohol wipes, bandages, tourniquets, dressings and equipment used in physical examination) is helpful in assisting both preschool and school age children dramatize the experiences in which they have had little control. The miniature hospital (containing nurses' station, nursery, semiprivate and multi-bed wards, bathroom, x-ray, treatment and anesthesia rooms) stimulates imaginative play where intense feelings are given expression. The child becomes the manipulator instead of the helpless victim; thus, turning passive experiences into action ones— the silent into the divulged in the process of mastery.

Many hospitals do not recognize the importance of sending children confined to beds, wheelchairs or stretchers to the play area. Even the debilitated can join some of the activities—to leave a child behind while others go off to play is obviously unfair.

Social, occupational and educational aspects of play are also planned. Arts, crafts, and music are part of the well-equipped playroom and can easily synchronize with the school program.

The best assurance that play needs will be met is through organized recreational programs. In institutions where they are not yet developed, the burden for play activities rests heavily with the nursing staff who have the greatest responsibility for the management of the child's daily activities. However, this means that play of necessity, becomes secondary to physical care; therefore, it is unlikely to achieve the importance it deserves.

Handling Feelings of Hostility and Aggression

Major physical hurt and loss of close relationships engender anger and anxiety shown in a multitude of ways. Especially vulnerable are children

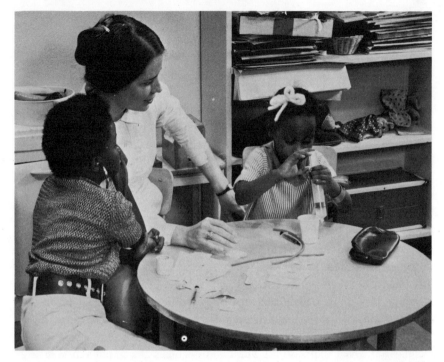

Fig. 5-5. A child's learning of nondestructive avenues of expression requires the guidance of understanding adults. Feelings are not resolved by denial or avoidance. (photo taken from the film "Play in the Hospital," Play School Association, Campus Films)

who already have disturbed relationships with the mother or those children who have been subject to family conflict. In situations where play is not a regular feature of the child's hospital life, the management of hostility and aggression may be a major problem. Destruction of property, kicking, biting, bullying and uncooperativeness are frequently manifestations. Children are disturbed in direct relationship to their instability prior to hospitalization.

Professionals need to know that not all children act out aggressive feelings, and that resentment emerges under permissive conditions. Where tight controls are maintained, children are not free to reveal themselves. It is more usual for a child to express negative feelings in an atmosphere of security.

Before pediatric personnel can deal with children's hostility constructively, its existence must be expected. Feelings are not resolved by denial and avoidance. The learning of nondestructive avenues of expression requires the guidance of understanding adults. Children who are permitted to dramatize and verbalize hostility can try new solutions to formerly unacceptable manifestations and thus achieve greater potential for adaptation.

Under no circumstances should the aggression of children be met with counter-aggression from professionals. Firmness is appropriate where a child needs controls but hostility from the staff will mean that they perceive the child as dangerous. This reaction in turn creates further misbehavior or withdrawal on the part of the child.

There are as many opportunities to handle aggression on the pediatric units as there are in the play areas. Medical personnel are in strategic positions to take care of problems on the spot; e.g., when Bill does not eat his dinner because his mother failed to show up during visiting hours; when Carol beats her doll after medication is forced on her; when Victor does not speak to his pediatrician because he was not discharged as anticipated.

> Several boys ranging from 4 to 7 years ganged up on the nurse passing medications. As she entered their room, they squirted her with carefully aimed syringes. She was startled at first but managed to maintain her composure. Expecting her to meet their aggression with the same, they began to flee until they realized she did not intend to retaliate. Instead, she surprised them by expressing sympathy for their feelings. "I suppose you're really angry with me for all the needles I've been giving you. I don't blame you." Her statement stimulated a barrage of feeling and opened discussions on why each was receiving intramuscular injections. She helped them to examine their reactions consciously.

The nature of aggression forces it to be recognized one way or another; this is true in family settings as well. However, the development of affection—the ability to love, is rarely if ever promoted in any setting. Why this is so may be due to the more threatening quality aggression has for its objects and the power it lends to the aggressor if not checked. Affection and tenderness can easily go unnoticed. The offerer of positive feelings is vulnerable to rejection and therefore is reticent.

As part of a therapeutic play program, evocation of hostility is therefore only half of the work. The staff must become attuned to the whisperings of tenderness, generosity and warmth that the children will make.[10] Role playing, particularly the nutritive aspects of doctoring and nursing, needs prominence once the hostility is evoked. To show the child how to be gentle toward a puppet or an animal shows him that grown-ups value these capacities that he can easily call forth in himself. A most skilled play session will leave the child aggressive in demanding and giving love. Again this program goes beyond the minimization of trauma and containment of children—it initiates and augments growth toward humaneness.

An individual's ability to encourage the expression of feeling in others depends to a great extent upon the tolerance of such feelings in himself. Staff members who cannot tolerate overt positive and negative feelings will find it difficult to allow them in children; with such people children would learn to conceal their reactions or develop guilt regarding them.

> A pediatric nurse reported that she found it necessary to stop a child's needle play because of the intensity of his reactions. "Adam jabbed the doll's head, abdomen and back repeatedly. The look of hatred on his face scared me. He wouldn't play nicely so I had to take away the equipment."

Needle Play

Injections, part of the treatment of almost all pediatric patients are universally feared. The importance of therapeutic play in this area cannot be overstressed. A child will interpret any sharp object stuck into his body as a brutal attack by a more powerful person.

Ideally, needle play follows immediately after and in-between the experience of having an injection (of all types). Most children get started with very little help, but the nurse, doctor or technician must be willing to supply equipment, supervision, and support in order to make this an interaction.

Having equipment easily available in a dramatic play equipment drawer on the units allows for spur of the moment action. Necessary props for I.M., I.V. and finger tip needle play are stuffed dolls or animals, alcohol wipes, clean syringes and needles, 30 cc. water vials labelled for dramatic play, miniature I.V. sets made with discarded I.V. tubing, clamps and small bottles, medicine cups, small tourniquets, tongue blades (for arm boards), blood tubes, adhesive tape and band-aids. Older children prefer withdrawing fluid from vials while younger children are more adept at drawing water into a syringe from a widemouthed container. Some patients may not want to give an injection to a favorite doll, but they accept substitutes easily.

To get started, a staff member may demonstrate the method of giving an injection. A child's attention is engaged by drawing up the solution and squirting a bit into the air. This demonstration is usually fascinating to the child and helps him to discover the non-painful aspects of injection. Then strict attention to the actual technique involves him in the procedure and makes him less fearful of the tools. While administering the injection, making appropriate expressions of distress for the doll teaches the child that crying and protests are permitted and that the giver realizes that needles hurt. A staff member playing the part of both the doll and nurse (or doctor) may ask why needles are necessary and then respond to his own questions in order to bring out some of the child's fantasies:

> Doll: "Ow, that hurts. Why do I have to get these awful shots?"
> Nurse: "I know it hurts. Help me by holding still so that I can finish quickly. I don't blame you for not liking it."
> Doll: "Don't do it, I'll be good."
> Nurse: "Oh, you don't know why you're getting this needle. You think you're being punished? Do you know what's in this syringe and what the medicine does?"
> Doll: "No, I don't." (Tearfully)
> Nurse: "This medicine will make you a bit sleepy before your operation just as I told you. Some children think they are being punished—but we don't do things like that here. When we don't like what children are doing, we tell them so and also what we expect. We never give needles to punish."

When a child refuses to participate, it is wise to tell him that he does not have to and to continue to play for him as a way of holding his interest. If he remains hesitant, pretend that it is too difficult to do it alone. Ask the child to place his hand on yours to help you draw up the water, later to push in the needle. Before long he should be working on his own with support. Another way to encourage a fearful child is to allow group dramatic play. It is a rare patient who is not caught up by the enthusiasm and confidence of peers. Allowing the child to keep a disposable syringe (without a needle) and other safe equipment permits him to practice afterwards without staff supervision. Just because a child appears comfortable with a group or parents does not mean that this is true when he is alone. Therefore after needle play of any sort, he needs to be checked to make sure he understands and integrates the experience. The older child (7 on) can have proportionately less play and more scientific explanation as to the usefulness of putting medicine directly into the body or taking blood samples out.

Parents approval of needle play insures that the child can participate comfortably. Frequently there is a fear that this play will stir up feelings and make the child violent. Explaining that the technique is a way of helping the child overcome his fears by making him familiar with the instrument and giving him an acceptable way to handle feelings may decrease parent resistance. However, when disapproval continues, it means

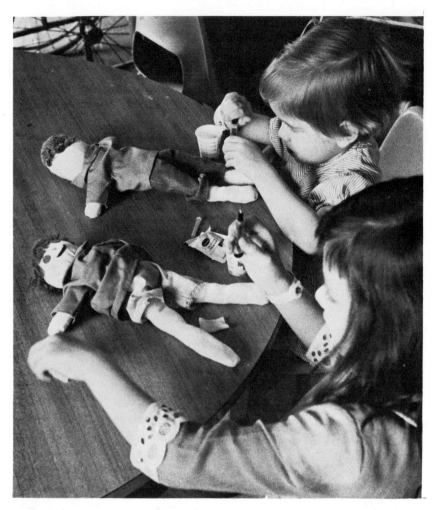

Fig. 5-6. One way to encourage a fearful child is to allow group dramatic play.
(photo by Hilary Smith)

that the child most likely will be unable to continue in his parent's presence.
(See Chapter 4.)

In summary, play is an effective means by which a puzzling and sometimes painful real world can be approached. When he can deal with things
that are small or inanimate the child masters situations that to him may
be otherwise overwhelming. By miniaturizing and experimenting with the
dangers from the external world of the hospital and the internal world of
his imagination, play strengthens the ego to more confidently adapt to and
solve future challenges.

REFERENCES

1. Erikson, E. H.: Studies in the interpretation of play. Genetic Psychology Monographs, *22*:561, 1940.
2. Axline, V.: Play Therapy: The Inner Dynamics of Childhood. p. 150. Boston, Houghton Mifflin Co., 1947.
3. Slavson, S.: Play group therapy for young children. The Nervous Child, *7*:320, 1948.
4. Rambert, M. L.: Graphic and plastic materials. *In* Haworth, M. R. (ed.): Child Psychotherapy: Practice and Theory. New York, Basic Books, 1964.
5. Freud, A.: Normality and Pathology in Childhood. p. 136. New York, International Universities Press, 1965.
6. Blumgart, E., and Korsh, B. M.: Pediatric recreation. An approach to meeting the emotional needs of hospitalized children. Pediatrics, *34*:133, 1964.
7. Plank, E. N.: Working with Children in Hospitals. Cleveland, The Press of Case-Western Reserve University, 1962.
8. Tisza, V. B., *et al.:* The use of a play program by hospitalized children. J. Amer. Acad. Child Psychiat., *19*:515, 1970.
9. Brooks, M.: Play for hospitalized children. Young Children, *24*: 224, 1969.
10. Josselyn, I. M.: The capacity to love: a possible reformulation. J. Amer. Acad. Child Psychiat., *10*:1, 1971.

BIBLIOGRAPHY

Adams, M. L., and Berman, D. C.: The hospital through a child's eyes. Children, *12*:102, 1965.

Frank, L. K.: Play in personality development. Amer. J. Orthopsychiat., *25*:576, 1955.

Hartley, R. E., Frank, L. K., and Goldenson R. M.: Understanding Children's Play. Chapters 1, 2, 3. New York, Columbia University Press, 1952.

Hellersberg, E. F., *et al.:* Developmental phases of play. *In* Haworth, M. R. (ed.): Child Psychotherapy: Practice and Theory. New York, Basic Books, 1964.

Jolly, H.: Play and the sick child. Lancet, *2*:1286, 1968.

Lowenfeld, M.: Play in Childhood. New York, John Wiley & Sons, 1967.

Read, K.: The Nursery School: A Human Relations Laboratory. ed. 3. Philadelphia, W. B. Saunders, 1960.

Redl, F., and Wineman, D.: The Aggressive Child. New York, The Free Press, 1957.

Tisza V. B., and Angoff, K.: A play program and its function in a pediatric hospital. Pediatrics, *19*:293, 1957.

6

Preparing Children and Parents for Diagnostic and Surgical Procedures

Teaching models for preparing children and parents for commonly encountered diagnostic and surgical procedures are presented on the following pages. These models were developed for use in a specific hospital and, therefore, will require some modification for use in other institutions.

The material is divided into 7 parts and is so arranged as to keep repetition at a minimum. Parts 2, 4, 5 and 6 are general and apply to all patients. Part 1 contains 6 subparts (A to F) that concern various age groups. Part 3, with 8 sections (A to H), deals with particular procedures.

Part 1. Guidelines for working with

    A. Newborns
    B. Infants
    C. Toddlers and Young Threes
    D. Older Threes- to Seven-Year-Olds
    E. Seven- to Thirteen-Year-Olds
    F. Adolescents

Part 2. Guidelines for Initiating Teaching When a Diagnostic or Surgical Procedure is Scheduled

Part 3. Preparation of a Child for
    A. Tonsillectomy
    B. Herniorrhaphy
    C. Eye Surgery
    D. Kidney Biopsy
    E. Urologic Surgery
    F. Cardiac Catheterization
    G. Cardiac Surgery
    H. Brain Surgery

Part 4. General Instructions for All Patients on the Day Before Treatment

Part 5. Instructions for All Patients on the Day of Surgery

Part 6. Helping the Child to Cope with Feelings Related to Hospitalization and Treatment: Post-Procedural Period

Part 7. Body Outlines Used for Children and Parents

Directions for use: Choose an age group and procedure listed above; for example, a 7-year-old to be prepared for cardiac surgery. Turn to the following sections: Part 1, E; Part 2; Part 3, G; Part 4; Part 5; and Part 6.

PART 1. A
GUIDELINES FOR WORKING WITH NEWBORNS

DIRECTIONS	COMMENTS
1. Assign one staff member to care for newborn.	Newborns have been found to distinguish between equally competent caretakers at 10 days of age.
2. Establish calm, quiet, comforting environment: a. subdued lighting b. soundproofing c. maintenance of constant warmth d. sure, gentle handling with tactile stimulation (closeness, holding, rocking and pacifiers when distressed)	From the moment of birth, the newborn is acutely aware of his surroundings. This includes sight, hearing, touch and temperature. The startle reflex of some newborns reveals those who have heightened sensitivities. An immediate response to alleviate distress is partly responsible for establishing basic trust. (See Chapter 2.)
3. Permit routines to be determined by the newborn: a. feeding b. diapering c. bathing d. sleeping e. examining	Each newborn is unique. It is inhumane to force artificial schedules based on the convenience of hospital shifts. Newborns will begin their own vegetative cycles if allowed to do so. These are noted in the first few weeks only by special measurements. However, unless the individual infant is allowed this freedom, later clinically apparent patterns are either made chaotic or permanently rigid. In particular, sleep cycles can be disrupted for months after too much time is spent in a brightly lit nursery. Examinations if timed when the newborn is awake, interfere least with the carefully established environment of security.
4. Explain to parents the rationale behind the nursery policies.	By instruction and example, parents will incorporate these tenets. They also have the leisure and freedom from the larger family to discuss doubts with their doctor or nurse.
5. Encourage rooming-in.	With rooming-in the mother has greater control of the environment and the opportunity to get to know her small infant. She

	is usually quite receptive to suggestions for handling and responding to the child's needs.
6. Develop classes for parents.	This will stimulate discussion of different infant care practices and family-cultural attitudes.

PART 1. B
GUIDELINES FOR WORKING WITH INFANTS

DIRECTIONS	COMMENTS
1. Assign one staff member and a relief person to care for child and to work with mother.	For this young group most of the staff's support is given to the mother so that she can continue mothering responsibilities under stress.
2. Make initial contacts with infant in mother's presence until he regards you as a safe person.	This is particularly important for infants over 5 months of age.
3. Interview parents for information on infant's routines. Incorporate what is appropriate into hospital schedule, allowing for flexibility.	The staff should inquire about eating habits, home routine and methods of comforting baby, so that the infant develops trust that needs will be met. During interview it is possible to pick up areas where parents need assistance with infant care.
4. Provide opportunity for parents to express feelings regarding the baby's illness and hospital experiences.	When parents are stifled, under stress they frequently find outlets by making the staff scapegoats or in becoming irritated with the child or each other.
5. Provide infant with tactile and sensory stimulation, also comfort and pleasure experiences.	The infant should be provided with singing, talking, music, mobiles, infant seats and swings, strollers, carriages, rockers, cuddling, security objects from home, hand toys. Comfort measures are especially important when the infant is denied food prior to a test or surgery.
6. Encourage mother to participate in the infant's care as much as possible.	It is important for a mother to feel comfortable with her sick child. Continuous contact facilitates this. Young babies know their mothers. When the mother's participation in care is not feasible, emphasize the importance of a regular visiting pattern. The closer the child is to the toddler age group, the more imperative mother's presence becomes, because this is the normal separation-individuation phase which requires mother's presence for success. Can rooming-in or rooming-by be arranged?

For infants, continuity of maternal care (on which emotional, social and intellectual growth is dependent) is of paramount importance. In the absence of a constant mother figure, arrange for a mother substitute. Staff needs to take responsibility for maintaining constancy of care. No 2 caretakers are the same and babies know this immediately.

7. Turn to Part 2 for further guidelines that can be applied to infants.

PART 1. C
GUIDELINES FOR WORKING WITH TODDLERS AND YOUNG THREES

DIRECTIONS	COMMENTS
1. Assign one person to care for child and to work with mother.	For this young group, most of the staff's support will be given to the mother so that she can continue mothering responsibilities under stress.
2. Interview parents for information on child's habits and routines. Incorporate what is appropriate into hospital schedule.	Provide potty chair when child is trained; if mother wishes a 2- or 3-year-old to have bottles, do not attempt to change his habits in the hospital. Allow nightlight if used at home.
3. Provide opportunities for parents to express feelings regarding child's illness and hospital experiences.	
4. Encourage mother to participate in her child's care and to see him frequently throughout the day.	The toddler group experiences the greatest amount of regression due to separation. Attachment to mother is very strong and the child's capacity for verbal expression is not yet well established. His chief preoccupations are abandonment and individuation.
	Is rooming-in or rooming-by feasible? Arrange for a mother substitute when a constant mothering figure is not available.
5. Give parents permission to leave their child and help in separating from him. Instruct them to indicate when they will return in relation to the child's activities, because time is not understood by this age group. Ask parents to leave personal articles with child to assure him of their return. Assist parents in leaving immediately after announcing	Many parents experience guilt when the child protests their leaving, and need extra support at these times. Some try "sneaking out" to avoid scenes. They must understand that such action impairs the child's trust in them. Clinging needs to be interpreted as separation anxiety which subsides when parents set up a pattern of reappearance and keep promises made to the child.

their departure. Stay with the child to help him over the difficult period.

6. Ask parents to bring in familiar toys and family photos. Make up stories involving pleasant home activities. Encourage parents to do the same.

Repeat effective stories again and again. This provides for stability when everything else appears to be changing for the child. Avoid stories with separation themes, unless they end with a reunion (for example, "King Midas and the Golden Touch"); they increase feelings of abandonment. Avoid fairy tales and analogies because this age group cannot distinguish fact from fiction, nor make comparisons. If child reveals fantasies, help him to end them happily.

7. Provide toddler with intellectual and motor stimulation.

8. Allow toddler to play with safe equipment used in his treatment.

The child should have the use of stethoscopes, reflex hammer, tongue blades, syringes without needles, dolls with appropriate attachments for a particular procedure.

9. When a treatment or surgery is scheduled, tell the toddler about it just before carrying it out. Verbal toddlers can be told the day before or early in the morning when surgery is to occur later in the day. Three-year-olds are told the day before or earlier if extensive preparation is required. Be truthful about hurting. Give permission to object but be positive about what you are doing. If there is no choice, do not imply there is by asking the child if you may proceed.

Telling about an event which then occurs builds confidence that the staff mean what they say.

10. Refrain from talking about a young child within his

A young child's capacity to understand far exceeds his capacity to verbalize. His hearing. Assume that he understands.

interpretations are literal. Choose words with care. See *Egocentric thinking,* page 23.

For the toddler and young 3-year-old, hospitalization is less of a devastating event when medical personnel understand the need for (1) continuity of the mother–child relationship, (2) the incorporation of familiar routines and rituals (when they are not in conflict with medical goals), (3) structure and limit setting, and (4) mastery and control.

11. Turn to Part 2 for further guidelines which can be applied to toddlers and young 3's.

PART 1. D
GUIDELINES FOR WORKING WITH OLDER THREES– TO SEVEN–YEAR–OLDS

DIRECTIONS	COMMENTS
1. Assign one nurse to the child as consistently as possible. Designate a relief person.	
2. Use a body outline, doll and other visual aids in teaching.	This age group is capable of understanding the inside of the body; so a simple explanation of anatomy and physiology is given and drawn in on the outline.
	A doll is used to visualize external appearance post-procedure or surgery (tubes, bandages, intravenous equipment). Toys or models representing equipment used in the child's care increase comprehension and are conducive to dramatic play. This age group is challenging to teach; 3- to 7-year-olds are highly imaginative and have developed communication skills which facilitate active participation in teaching.
	Encourage child's questions and compliment his inquisitiveness. Give him credit for understanding. Maximize initiative and mastery in order to increase the child's pride in himself.
3. Deal with the castration and mutilation fantasies common to this age group (phallic phase) by talking of damage and repair.	See example of restitutive play in the story of Robinson, page 221.
4. Reassure child repeatedly, whenever appropriate, that no one is to blame for his condition or hospitalization, and that the procedures are limited.	Although this is recommended in all teaching, it is especially important for 3- to 7-year-olds who are preoccupied with guilt and blame. The child tends to generalize and feels that all body parts are vulnerable.
5. For 3 and 4-year-olds, encourage mother's participation in the child's care.	This tells the child that mother approves of hospital routines and helps the child to integrate concepts of body care.

6. Impress mother with the importance of a regular visiting pattern.

A pattern of visiting builds confidence in her return. From 3 to 4 years, ambivalence is characteristic, as demonstrated in alternating behavior: expression of love and hate, defiance and compliance, clinging and independence.

7. For 5-year olds, encourage participation in medical care and self-hygiene.

For this age; self-care has just been accomplished; thus, it is threatening to relinquish it to others. The child tends to be upset by smells and messiness as he has just achieved bowel and bladder control and learned prohibitions against dirt. He needs to participate in cleaning up. Responsibility for self-care also includes the avoidance of unnecessary risks and the knowledge of safety equipment on the unit.

8. Observe for evidence of silent attachment to the staff. This positive sign from the

For 3- to 7-year-olds, the staff needs to be aware of the development of oedipal attachments, that is, girls may become

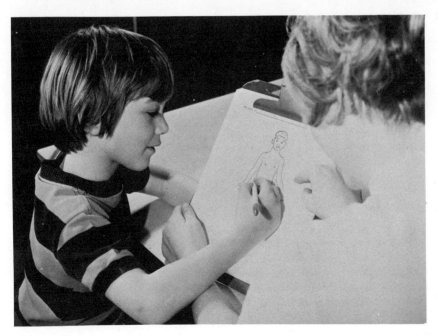

Fig. 6-1. An explanation of anatomy and physiology is given and drawn in on the body outline after determining the child's understanding of his illness. (photo by Steve Campus)

child can be openly recognized and appropriately supported.

flirtatious or silent with male personnel. Boys may show sexual curiosity overtly or covertly toward female personnel. Boys and girls may compete with one another to win the favor of the secretly loved adult. To have a warm response from an esteemed and favored grown-up may further healthy identification and build confidence the child this age needs to enter latency competitions: physically, socially and academically.

9. Turn to Part 2 for further guidelines which can be applied to 3- to 7-year-olds.

PART 1. E
GUIDELINES FOR WORKING WITH SEVEN– TO THIRTEEN–YEAR–OLDS

DIRECTIONS	COMMENTS
1. Assign one person to care for child consistently. Designate a relief person.	
2. Teach child scientific terminology for body parts and medical procedures after learning his words for them.	This age group is interested in a scientific approach.
3. Determine whether a doll is to be used in teaching.	Some children ask for them while others are embarrassed to be seen with dolls. If used, the doll can be called a dummy or teaching doll. When postoperative appearance is difficult to describe, visualization on a dummy is recommended.
4. Continue with the use of body outlines for explanation of anatomy and physiology and visualization of postoperative appearance.	
5. Be straightforward about telling the child that no other part of the body will be involved—only the operative area described.	If a child is immature for his age or preoccupied with mutilation, follow directions for the under 7 group.
6. Encourage questioning, expression of feelings and active participation in his teaching.	Although the teaching plan is similar to that of younger children, the response of 7- to 13-year-olds is usually more enthusiastic. In relating to this age level we can take advantage of the characteristics already developed: the ability to reason, to make generalizations and to understand the concept of time.
	Generally, these children have fewer adjustment problems due to hospitalization. They are able to tolerate separation from parents; they are interested in developing relationships outside of the family and enjoy sharing experiences with their peer

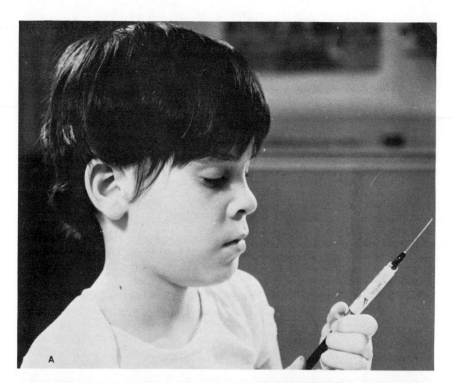

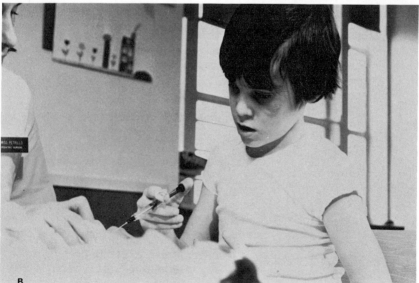

Fig. 6-2 A-D. This sequence illustrates the lessening of a child's anxiety through participation in preoperative dramatic play. By the last photo, we see the beginning of a sense of confidence. (photos by Steve Campus)

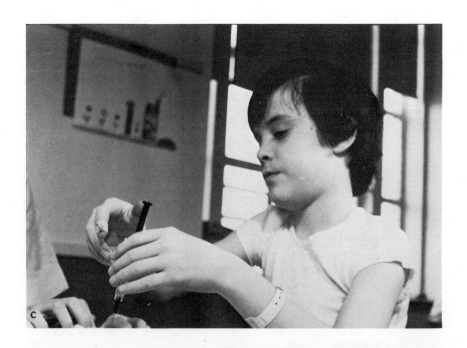

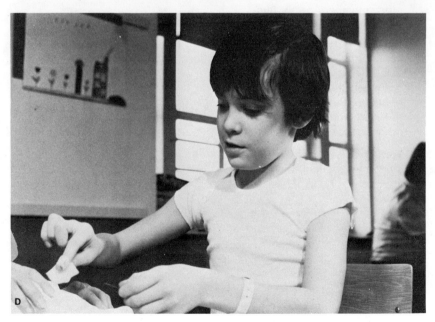

Figure 6-2 (*Continued*)

group. Hospitalization can become an educational and social experience providing the preparation is adequate. The group is more reality-oriented and capable of learning a great deal from contacts with the staff and other children. Teaching and management are easier because these children can verbalize feelings, comprehend cause and effect, and have a scientific orientation.

A regressed child of this age group may fear mutilation, monsters and separation. Fear of death is common at this period; not infrequently a child will ask directly if he is going to die, or tell stories of children who have had complicated illnesses.

7. Beware of reassuring a child about his condition before eliciting his notion of what is wrong and how it happened. Then get his experiences with illness and hospitalization, and of other members of his family and friends.

This is important in order to emphasize the differences and similarities between his problem and those of others. This can be most reassuring. Despite the reality-orientation of this group, one must be alert to misconceptions about illness.

It is also helpful to express confidence in his doctor and in a staff that is well trained in the management of his problem and to mention the numbers of children successfully treated.

Children here can comprehend simple statistical probability. (See Chapter 2.)

8. Turn to Part 2 for further guidelines which may be applied to 7- to 13-year-olds.

PART 1. F
GUIDELINES FOR WORKING WITH ADOLESCENTS

DIRECTIONS	COMMENTS
1. Assign one nurse to care for the patient consistently. Designate a relief person.	The nurse assigned should not be close to adolescence herself. Ideally, she should be a mature, consistent but flexible individual who has understanding of her own behavior.
2. Plan teaching for periods when parents are absent. Make provision to see the parents at another time.	It is difficult for the adolescent to confide in his nurse or doctor in the presence of his parents. Respect his need for privacy.
3. Discover the words he uses for body parts. Then, teach him scientific terms for gaps in his knowledge.	Medical terminology will be readily absorbed into his vocabulary.
4. Encourage him to ask questions.	It will be easier for him to approach the staff when he has the verbal tools. Tell him that most patients think of questions later on and that he probably will also.
	Characteristically, the adolescent is preoccupied about physical changes and having a body that is different from others. He is curious about sex and may give the impression of knowing more or less than he actually does know. A trusting atmosphere may lead to sex education opportunities. The staff should be receptive and informative.
	Castration anxiety shows itself at this stage by concern about body size, secondary sexual development, and in a boy's hostility toward girls or in a girl's denial of femininity.
5. Reassure the patient that his questions and your conversations are confidential.	The only time a confidence cannot be respected is when it places the patient in jeopardy. In such an instance, tell the patient this.
6. Determine whether the teen-ager has done reading about his disease or condition. If the patient	

is concerned about genetic factors in his disease or condition, arrange for genetic counseling.

7. Use a body diagram to give a scientific explanation of the anatomy and physiology involved in his surgery or procedure.

Often medical personnel credit the adolescent with understanding that he does not have. His misconceptions need clarification. He may have vague ideas about body function which remain unclear because he is embarrassed to ask or does not have the ability to make his needs known. He may need help in doing so, but he is capable of abstract thinking and learning on a sophisticated level.

8. Include patient in conferences with family and medical-nursing team to discuss plans for his treatment.

The adolescent patient wants to be in on the planning, although sometimes he prefers not to know when findings are too threatening. Thus, do not invariably give direct answers to questions before checking out the purpose of the question.

9. Provide for continuation of social activities and mature identifications.

The child should have telephone facilities and opportunities to visit outside of the hospital when confinement is lengthy. Teen recreation program, peer relationships from the patient population and peer visiting should be allowed. Encourage patients to assist with younger children and clerical activities.

10. Arrange for diet preferences (when medically sound).

Teen-agers enjoy being able to prepare their own food and snacks.

11. Arrange for continuing education (hospital school or tutor) when illness is prolonged.

Intellectual talk may be a useful way to start a relationship.

12. Determine rules and regulations for teen-agers on the unit or for an adolescent unit. Make information available to staff and patients, preferably in writing.

Early Adolescence

Characteristically during this phase there is a withdrawal of interest in the original love objects as the adolescent makes initial attempts at emancipation from the family. The use of hostility, provocative behavior, questioning of traditional values, secretiveness and vacillation between dependent and independent attitudes (as measures for loosening ties) is strong and may be manifested also in relationships to authority figures (such as hospital personnel) as well as with parents. He may be antisocial or delinquent. Before new love relationships can be established, the adolescent experiences loneliness and depression resulting in much self-preoccupation. Self-focus increases with illness to the point, at times, or hypochondriasis.

13. Talk to the youngster about his body if he seems comfortable.

14. It is useful for the staff to be more personal about how they chose their vocations.

A hospitalization at this time may influence the teen-ager to seriously consider a health career (formation of new ego ideal).

15. Beware of being drawn in on the child's anger toward the family. Empathize with difficulties and infatuations but avoid identifying (allowing self to take on the adolescent's hostilities and yearnings).

Middle Adolescence

Alienation from parents prevails. The adolescent relies heavily upon the peer group. However, now he has acquired some sense of self and is capable of seeking out new love objects. Mourning and being in love are typical moods. Introspective daydreaming often helps to relieve feelings of isolation until a close tie is established with the opposite sex. Heterosexual love objects vary: they either strongly resemble or are completely different from the parent of the opposite sex. Although sudden attachments or hostilities to hospital personnel may appear to be unfounded, they are actually of much relevance to understanding the dynamics of behavior and in understanding the adolescent's vulnerability to rejection. Provision needs to be made for consistency in relationships to key people throughout hospitalization.

Intense feelings are common as is intellectualization to avoid the same unmanageable feelings. There is the tendency to asceticism in order to bolster the denial of unacceptable feelings; e.g., the welcoming of tribulation and pain. Loneliness is countered by self-stimulation—masturbation, the taking of physical risks, the use of drugs. Consequently, the adolescent may be prone to addiction, especially if it is a fad of the peer group.

Late Adolescence

In this phase, the adolescent is capable of mature, logical reflection. He evaluates his ideals, strengths, aspirations and thinks in terms of the future—of a life plan. The conflict between dependence and independence is resolved. He is emancipated from his parents and from the peer group as well. It is a period of consolidation, of acceptance and of coming to grips with feelings.

In the hospital, the adolescent girl reacts to illness by showing concern for appearance—by giving attention to the whole body. Treatment is viewed in terms of how it will affect relationships with boys and the reproductive process.

16. Be reasonably complimentary. The teen-ager deserves credit for being stoical in the face of the humiliation illness imposes.

The adolescent boy shows concern about virility and prowess, and how mutilation of the body will affect his abilities. The self-image is threatened for both sexes. They are future-oriented in relation to the opposite sex and vocational choice. They need all the support the staff can realistically give in these areas.

A chronic or severe illness in adolescence may interfere with any or all the major developmental goals for this period—emancipation from the family, heterosexual attachments, management of feelings, and preparation for a vocation.

17. Turn to Part 2 for further guidelines which can be applied to adolescents.

PART 2

GUIDELINES FOR INITIATING TEACHING WHEN A DIAGNOSTIC OR SURGICAL PROCEDURE IS SCHEDULED

DIRECTIONS	COMMENTS
1. After referring to Part 1 for information on preparing a specific age group, you are ready to initiate teaching. Assign one person to carry out preparation and a relief person.	Consistency in relationships will facilitate the development of the child's trust in the teacher. For most hospitals, at present, the nursing staff is in the best position to follow through on teaching and dramatic play. It is practical to have this aspect of the program organized under one discipline. The participation of other professional staff, however, is to be encouraged.
2. Consult with pediatrician or surgeon regarding the plan of treatment and the information given to the parents.	
3. Review the parents' understanding of what is going to take place and how they have explained it to their child. What terms were used? What symptoms did the child exhibit at home? How were they related to the child's condition?	This information will indicate how much additional help the child and his parents will need and the direction the teaching should take.
4. Determine whether the parents are to participate in the teaching or whether they should be present. See Parent Participation, page 73.	When parents are cooperative and supportive to the child, their presence in teaching sessions is desirable. Otherwise plan separate sessions for parents and child.
5. Decide appropriate explanation for age and emotional maturity and choose vocabulary suitable to child's intellectual understanding. Use neutral words like opening, drainage and oozing instead of cut and bleed.	Neutral words are less likely to frighten the child and allow him to control going into more dangerous connotations or holding to harmless meanings.

6. Gather all visual aids and dramatic play materials to be used.

Having a supply of teaching aids and dramatic play materials prepared in advance in a designated place makes it easier to proceed; e.g., body outlines, dolls, drainage tubing, model I.V. equipment, bandages, syringes and needles, anesthesia mask, model of croupette made out of plastic bag, and even models of frequently used machines.

7. Plan to cover the entire teaching in approximately 3 sessions.

Even when time is limited, this allows the child to assimilate the material and to ask questions. Too much at one time overwhelms him and he is likely to "tune out." Moreover, focus is lost with a greater number of sessions. Ideally, children are admitted a minimum of 2 days in advance of major surgery so that adequate time is available to the staff.

8. Make a sketchy outline for each session and refer to it to assure complete coverage.

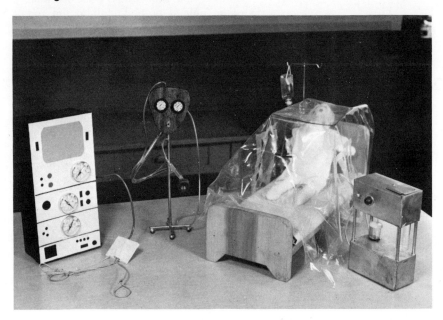

Fig. 6-3. Having a supply of visual aids and dramatic play materials makes it easier to proceed with preoperative teaching. (photo by Steve Campus)

9. Before giving the child any information, determine his understanding of the problem and the reason for hospitalization.

This frequently discloses fantasies which might be missed if teaching is started immediately. His answers will indicate the emphasis of your teaching and the kind of reassurances needed.

When a child denies any knowledge, do not take this at face value. He may be hoping that through denying the event, it will not take place. Ask him instead, "How did you know that you needed to come to the hospital? What did the doctor say? What did mother and father tell you?" If he still professes ignorance, try this approach. "I guess you must be wondering what it's all about. Naturally you can't know if your ideas are right, but tell me what things have come to your mind." Or, "You can't possibly know since you haven't been in this situation before. Are you the kind of person who lets things happen without asking? If I were you, I'd like to know. I don't like surprises."

Another approach would be to tell a story of an animal or child left in the repair shop to have something fixed.

10. Turn now to Part 3 for specific information on preparing a patient for a procedure or surgery.

PART 3. A
PREPARATION OF A CHILD FOR TONSILLECTOMY

DIRECTIONS	COMMENTS AND EXAMPLES

1. Refer to Parts 1 and 2 before continuing.

2. After determining the child's understanding for hospitalization, give him a simple explanation to reinforce his knowledge or to correct his misunderstanding. Introduce symptoms.

"Tonsils are 2 small lumps in the back of your throat (or mouth). When you were smaller your tonsils helped to keep you from getting sick with sore throats, earaches and colds. But now, your tonsils are not working well. In fact, they are causing trouble by giving you earaches, sore throats and colds (whatever applies), and we know that's no fun. Your doctor can help. Because you don't need your tonsils anymore, they are going to be taken out. That's the reason you came to the hospital."

3. Reassure the child that no one is to blame for his condition. Make it clear that nothing he did is responsible.

4. Indicate postoperative expectations:
   a. sore throat
   b. ice collar
   c. medication
   d. positioning and emesis of old blood
   e. food and fluid restriction.

"When you wake up from your operation, your throat will feel quite sore. But we can make it feel better by putting an ice collar around your neck." (Show him an ice collar; open the top and indicate where the ice goes in. Allow him to try it on. Emphasize the coolness.) "And if it is necessary we can give medicine too."

"You will be placed on your belly because it will be easier for you to spit up old blood and phlegm that way. There will probably be a bit of old blood in your nose too. This usually happens. We expect it."

"In about 2 hours after returning to your room, you'll be ready to have something to drink. First we'll give you some cool ginger ale, because it will feel good. And later you may have some juices like apricot and pear. By tomorrow morning, you'll be ready for ice cream for breakfast, and that will feel good too. By then, you will be much better and you'll be able to go home. Your throat will still be sore, but every day it will feel better and soon you will feel fine again."

5. Ask child to show you the operative site on a body outline.

This frequently reveals confusion.

6. Reassure child that no other part of the body will be operated upon.

Use playful repetition to clarify operative area for child under 6. (See page 11.) Older children may be told directly.

7. Introduce needle play related to blood work already experienced.

This is introduced at the end of the session, because it is quite stimulating for the child. We want to be sure of his attention to the preceding material first.

Allow needle play. See Needle Play, page 130.

8. Play up rewards — how much he will have to tell his family and friends about the hospital, the new things he has seen, the different people he has met.

This allows the memory of stressful procedures to be associated with bravery and the wish for good health.

9. Turn to Part 4.

PART 3. B
PREPARATION OF A CHILD FOR HERNIORRHAPHY

DIRECTIONS	COMMENTS AND EXAMPLES

1. Refer to Parts 1 and 2 before continuing.

2. After determining child's fantasy regarding illness and hospitalization, give him a simple explanation of the anatomy and physiology involved, introducing symptoms.

Toddlers to Young 3's: "The doctor is going to fix this bump." (Indicate area on child and doll.) "He will do a little operation."

Older 3's to 7 Group:

"Have you heard about muscles? Show me one (biceps). Muscles are the parts of the body which allow you to move your arms and legs. Muscles also help to keep your back straight and your belly flat and firm. For some reason we don't know, your muscle here, . . ." (indicate on drawing) ". . . isn't as strong as it needs to be. Many are born this way, but, your doctor knows how to make the muscle stronger and tighter so that the bump will no longer be there. To do this he needs to do a small operation. The doctor will make a little opening here . . ." (draw in on outline) ". . . so that he can reach the muscle to be fixed."

7 Years and Older:

Same as above.

3. Reassure child that no one is to blame for his condition. Make it clear that nothing he has done contributed to it.

This is especially important for the 3 to 7 group because guilt regarding illness is a paramount feature.

4. Indicate postoperative appearance:
   a. sutures
   b. bandage
   c. intravenous infusion (not usually done for infants and toddlers)

"After the doctor fixes the muscle, he sews the opening with little black stitches, like this." (Draw on outline or doll.) "Over the spot he places a big bandage to keep the spot clean and to protect it."

(If appropriate) "You will also have a little tube in your arm that is attached to a bottle of sugar water. This is the way we feed children after an operation, until they are ready to eat again. This is to keep your stomach from getting upset."

5. Ascertain the child's understanding of your explanation by asking him simple questions and allowing him to place equipment on doll (bandage, I.V.) or to draw in answers on outline.

   Tell him he may ask questions at any time; in fact many children do.

Use a doll for toddlers; a doll and outline for the 3 to 7 group; an outline for 7 years and above. As the child permits, his own body may be used.

6. Reassure child that no other part of the body will be operated upon.

Use playful repetition to clarify operative area for children under 6. (See page 11.) Older children are told directly.

7. Introduce needle play related to blood work already experienced.

This is introduced at the end of the session, because it is quite stimulating for the child. We want to be sure of his attention to the preceding material first. See Needle Play, page 130.

8. Play up rewards — how much he will have to tell his family and friends about the hospital, the new things he has seen, the many people he has met.

This allows the memory of stressful procedures to be associated with bravery and the wish for good health.

9. Turn to Part 4.

PART 3. C
PREPARATION OF A CHILD FOR EYE SURGERY (STRABISMUS)

DIRECTIONS	COMMENTS AND EXAMPLES
1. Refer to Parts 1 and 2 before continuing.	
2. After determining the child's understanding of his condition and the reason for hospitalization, give him a simple explanation to reinforce his ideas or to correct his misunderstanding. Introduce symptoms.	*Toddlers to Young 3's:* "The doctor is going to straighten your eyes." *Older 3's to 7 Group:* "Do you know about muscles?" (Point to arm and leg.) "They are the parts of the body that allow you to move. Some muscles are large, like those in your arms and legs; there are small muscles too, like the ones that move your eyes. We know that the muscles of each eye are not working together; one eye turns in (or out) and the eyes don't line up together. And you say that you see double." (if it applies) "The reason for this is that the muscles for each eye are not the same size. We don't know why this is true; some children are probably born that way. Your doctor knows how to fix the muscles so that they can work together." *7 Years and Older:* In addition to above: "The unequal size and strength of the muscles cause a greater pull in one direction. This pull has happened to one eye (both eyes)."
3. Reassure child that no one is to blame for his condition. Make it clear that nothing he has done has contributed to it.	
4. Indicate the postoperative expectations: a. bandages over one or both eyes	Some surgeons will eliminate patches altogether. When both eyes are to be bandaged, it is important to arrange in advance for the continuous presence of a family member.

b. recognition of people by voice

c. member of family or nurse will be nearby to read to him, feed him, play music, keep him safe and tell him what is going on

d. wrist restraints to help him remember to keep hands away from eyes (when he is not constantly attended or when he dozes)

5. Ascertain the child's understanding of your explanation by asking simple questions and allowing him to place equipment on a doll. Indicate that you expect him to have questions and that he may ask at any time.

Familiarize the child with eye patches, restraints. Also play at recognizing voices and events in room with eyes closed.

6. Reassure child that no other part of the body will be operated upon.

Use playful repetition to clarify operative area for children under 6; older children may be told directly. (See page 11.)

7. Introduce needle play regarding blood work already experienced.

This is introduced at the end of the session, because it is quite stimulating for the child. We want to be sure of his attention to the preceding material first.

See Needle Play, page 130.

8. Play up rewards — how much he will have to tell his family and friends about his hospital experiences, the new things he has seen, and the new people he has met.

This allows the memory of stressful procedures to be associated with bravery and the wish for good health.

9. Turn to Part 4.

PART 3. D

PREPARATION OF A CHILD FOR A CLOSED KIDNEY BIOPSY

DIRECTIONS	COMMENTS AND EXAMPLES

1. Refer to Parts 1 and 2 before continuing.

2. After determining the child's fantasy regarding illness and hospitalization, give a simple explanation of the anatomy and physiology of the urinary system, using a body outline for a child over 3½.

Toddlers and Young 3's:

"The doctor is going to do a test to find out how to make you feel better. This is the place where the test will be." (Point to area.) Continue to focus on the outside of the body and external events.

Older 3's to 7 Group:

"You haven't heard of the word kidney before? Well, I'm not surprised; many boys and girls haven't. Let me draw them in on this picture of a boy (girl) I have brought for you. Kidneys are shaped like large beans, like this." (Draw kidneys in.) "There are two of them. Can you guess what kidneys do? It's their job to make urine. What do you call urine—wee wee, sisy, tinkle? When urine is made, it passes along these tubes coming from the kidneys and goes into a part called the bladder, where it collects. The bladder looks like a balloon; when it's full of urine, it's large. When you urinate (make wee wee) the urine comes out of the penis (or little opening between your legs), and the bladder empties."

7 Years and Older Group:

Grown-up terms such as ureters and urine are used and childish jargon and analogies are eliminated. In addition, a more scientific explanation is understood: "The work of the kidneys is to purify the blood by filtering (straining) the blood as it constantly passes through the kidneys. The kidneys hold back the parts of the blood that your body needs and allow water and waste products to pass off as urine. That's why your doctor does blood and urine tests; so he knows how well the kidneys are doing their job."

3. Introduce the child's symptoms and explain them in relation to the diagnostic procedure for the child over 3½.

"You seem to understand how the kidneys work. Remember the reasons your doctor brought you to the hospital; e.g., fever, puffiness, elevated blood pressure. These things gave your doctor the idea that your kidneys are not working as well as they could. So the doctor wants to do a test to find out exactly what the problem is. To do this, he needs to look at a tiny part of the kidney under a microscope. (That's a machine that makes things look much bigger than they are.) Once the doctor knows how the kidneys are working, he can decide how to help you get well."

4. Explain kidney biopsy in terms of specific steps:
   a. place for test
   b. x-ray table
   c. blood pressure cuff
   d. intravenous infusion

"You are probably wondering how this test is done. For this test, you will go to the x-ray room. Do you remember having an x-ray before?" (Recall details; show picture of an x-ray machine.) "You will be placed on the x-ray table, which has a camera overhead. All during the test, a blood pressure cuff will be around one arm. On the other arm, the doctor will start an intravenous infusion—that's an IV; a small tube will be put into your arm and a bottle of sugar water will be attached to it. This tube will be in place for a few hours, even after you get back to your room."

   e. personnel and attire

"Several people will be there with you; some you already know—your doctors, a nurse and the man or woman who takes the pictures. They will be wearing caps, masks, gowns and gloves."

   f. positioning

"You will be placed on the table like this —on your tummy with this small blanket roll under your belly." (Demonstrate with child on bed, placing the roll under the lower abdomen.) "This is done to raise your hips and to make it easier for the doctor to find the right spot to do the test. Where did I say the kidneys are? What do the kidneys do?"

g. draping and skin preparation

"Once you are in position, one doctor puts on gloves and cleans your skin with a special medicine on one side only, and then places towels around the spot where the test is going to be done. The reason for this is to make sure everything stays clean."

h. local anesthesia

"To make sure that you do not feel the test, the doctor will put some medicine into your skin with a tiny needle. You will know it; it will feel like a pinch, but you will feel nothing after that except pressure."

i. obtaining a specimen

"Right after this the doctor is ready to take a small piece of kidney—just a tiny amount, like a grain of rice—with a special instrument which is used for this. You won't feel any hurt, but you may feel the doctor's hand pressing on your side. It's uncomfortable but it's supposed to feel that way."

j. fluoroscopy

"While the test is going on, the x-ray man or lady will be taking pictures of your kidney. This is done to help the doctor find the best spot. In order to take these pictures, the room needs to be almost dark."

k. blood pressure readings

"While the doctors are doing the test, the nurse will be taking your blood pressure quite often. She will also be reminding you of what is going on. You may want to ask her questions."

l. bandage

"After the doctors take a tiny piece of kidney, the test is over. A small bandage will be placed over the spot to make sure it stays clean and protected."

End Session here; resume after an interval.

5. Review material covered in previous session. Evaluate how much has been retained. Ask child if he has thought of any questions since you spoke to him.

6. Explain routine following the test.

"When the test is over, you will return to your own room and this is what you can expect:

a. bed rest on your back for about 24 hours (a whole day);

b. frequent taking of your blood pressure, temperature and pulse;

c. collection of all urine for 24 hours;

d. intravenous for a few hours;

e. regular meals."

7. Explain preparation prior to procedure:

a. fasting

"When you go to bed this evening, we will place a tag on your bed that says NOTHING BY MOUTH. Because you will be getting medicine before your test, we don't want you to have anything to eat or drink during the night and in the morning. This is so your stomach will not become upset."

b. pre-procedure medication

"During the test it is important to stay in the position I described to you." (Remind child.) "In order to help you do this and so you won't mind the test too much, we will give you some medicine to make you drowsy. It has to be given by a small needle. I'll show you how it is done on this doll."

Demonstrate and allow needle play. See Needle Play, page 130.

8. Reassure child that no other part of the body will be involved.

Use playful repetition to clarify operative area for children under 6. (See page 11.) Older children may be told directly.

9. Ascertain child's understanding of your explanation by asking him simple questions in relation to the

Some children will not be able to verbalize answers but are able to playact or draw in answers on diagram.

diagram or doll. Allow him to reenact the procedure —attaching equipment, positioning doll, and taking a specimen.

10. Tell child that you will be with him during the procedure (if true) and that he will be taken in his bed (or stretcher) to the x-ray room.

This can be one of the most supportive measures we can provide. It can be managed when planned in advance.

11. Play up some of the rewards — that he will be seeing many new things and meeting many different people; that he will have a great deal to tell his family and friends about how big the x-ray machine was, how the doctors and nurses were dressed, how lights went on and off.

This allows the memory of stressful procedures to be associated with bravery and the wish for good health.

12. Delete Part 4; turn to Part 5.

PART 3. E

PREPARATION OF A CHILD FOR UROLOGIC SURGERY
(Repair of Bladder–Neck Obstruction and Reimplantation of One Ureter)

DIRECTIONS	COMMENTS AND EXAMPLES
1. Refer to Parts 1 and 2 before continuing.	
2. After determining the child's fantasy regarding illness and hospitalization, give him a simple explanation of the anatomy and physiology involved.	See explanation under Kidney Biopsy, page 165.
3. Introduce symptoms in relation to anatomy and physiology for child over 3½.	"You have already told me that you came to the hospital because of fevers and trouble making urine. There's a reason for this. I've told you how the kidneys, ureters (tubes) and bladder look and work." (Refer to drawing.) "This is the way it's supposed to be, but for some reason we don't understand, yours looks like this. This part of the bladder has a very small opening, so the urine (wee wee) cannot pass out easily; and this ureter (tube) is attached to the bladder higher up than it should be (or has a narrow part). It makes it hard for the urine to flow out. This is why sometimes the urine backs up, presses on the kidney, hurts, or causes fever. We know this because of the tests you have had (I.V.P., cystogram) and by the way you have been feeling."
4. When symptoms are absent, modify the approach.	"Although you haven't felt sick, the doctor knows that your kidneys, ureters and bladder are not working as they should because of the tests he has done and the examination he gave you in his office (clinic). He took your blood pressure, made x-ray pictures and did urine tests. The doctor knows that if this problem is not taken care of now, you may be sick later on."

5. Reassure the child that no one is to blame for his condition, and that nothing he has done contributed to it.

"We don't know why this is so. It's the way some are born. No one's to blame. It's certainly not because of anything you have done. But your doctor knows how to fix the parts—to make both these parts bigger so that the urine can pass through without any trouble. That's why you are going to have an operation."

Avoid specific details of the operative procedure. "The doctor will make an opening here so that he can reach the parts to be fixed." Draw in on diagram or doll.

6. Indicate postoperative appearance on drawing for child over 3½. For child under 3½, talk about external appearance on doll:

   a. urinary drainage tubing and collection bags

"After the doctor fixes the tube and bladder, he wants the parts to rest so that they will heal (get better) fast. To help do that, he puts in tubes in 3 parts. They are placed like this: one high in the ureter, one in the ureter lower down, and one in the bladder." (Draw in.) "This means that the urine will drain off without touching the parts that have been fixed."

"You won't be urinating (making wee wee) for a while. The urine will pass through the tubes into collection bags." (Draw in.) "At first the urine looks dark, then it becomes pink and finally yellow again. Sometimes you may feel like passing urine, but you won't NEED to."

   b. sutures
   c. bandage

"After the drainage tubes are in, the doctor closes the opening with little stitches and then places a large bandage over the spot. After the parts get better (heal) the doctor will take out the tubes, probably one at a time. Later he will take out stitches. We will show you how when it's about to happen."

   d. intravenous infusion

"After your operation, you won't be eating or drinking right away. We don't want to upset your stomach. So, instead of feeding you, we will give you sugar water through a tube in your arm." (Draw in.) "When you are ready to start eating again, we will start by giving you sips of water and juice first."

e. croupette

"Very often after operations, we place children in small plastic tents. You have probably seen them already. This helps them to breathe well and to keep cool. You will have one too." Show child a croupette or model of one.

7. Ascertain child's understanding of your explanation by asking simple questions regarding the drawing. Help him attach I.V. equipment, tubes, bandages to a doll.

Some children will not be able to verbalize answers to questions but may be able to point to or draw in answers on a diagram or playact their understanding.

8. Reassure child that no other part of the body will be operated upon.

Use playful repetition to clarify operative area for child under 6. (See page 11.) Older child may be told directly.

9. Play up rewards—that he will be seeing many new things and meeting different people; that he will have a great deal to tell his friends and family about the operation; that he will be able to explain it all with his diagram or doll.

This allows the memory of stressful procedures to be associated with bravery and the wish for good health.

10. Introduce needle play regarding blood work already experienced. Demonstrate and allow practice.

This is introduced at the end of the session so that it does not distract from the preceding material.

See Needle Play, page 130.

11. Continue with Part 4 after an interval.

PART 3. F
PREPARATION OF A CHILD FOR CARDIAC CATHETERIZATION

DIRECTIONS	COMMENTS
1. Refer to Parts 1 and 2 before continuing.	
2. After determining child's understanding of hospitalization, clarify or reinforce his understanding by discussing tests and visits to the cardiologist that may have occurred in the past —relating these to his present admission.	Most children have had ECG's and chest x-rays or may remember the doctor listening to the chest and heart. Some may know they have a murmur; others may have overheard adults talking about them and consequently have more knowledge than parents believe.
3. If the child has symptoms, explain that they are indications to the doctor that his heart may not be working as well as it could. Reassure child that no one is responsible for his condition.	
4. Explain to child that he needs to have a special test and pictures of his heart so that the doctor can discover the problem and also how to treat it.	
5. If a child is asymptomatic, discuss with him how the doctor became aware that his heart might not be working as well as it should. Then explain that the test and pictures will help determine if he has a problem with his heart.	For example, tell the child that the doctor listened to his chest and heard a murmur. Allow him to use a stethoscope.
6. Explain that he will be taken to a special place called the cardiac catheterization room.	

7. Describe how people will be dressed.

8. Explain that he will be lying on a moveable table, and that ECG leads will be placed on his arms and legs.

Recall other experiences with ECG's.

9. Tell child that his arms and legs will be loosely restrained.

"The loose ties around your arms and legs help you to remember to keep them in one place; so that you won't move about."

10. Explain that the nurse who is there inserts a rectal thermometer and leaves it in place throughout the test, so that she will know his temperature.

11. Explain that the doctor will wash the arm or groin, and put some medicine into the skin with a small needle. It will feel like a pinch, but thereafter he will not feel any pain (hurt). After the medicine, the doctor will make a small opening and insert a tiny tube.

Use a patient doll for toddlers, a doll and outline for 3½ to 6 year olds and an outline for older children to indicate the place where the tube will be inserted.

End session here. Resume after an interval.

12. Ask child simple questions to ascertain his understanding of the preceding material. Correct as necessary.

13. Describe atmosphere:

    a. noise and talk

"One machine will be making a humming sound all during the test."

"Some machines make clicking sounds."

"People talk a lot—mostly about their work."

"Sometimes the doctor will ask you questions."

"Sometimes you will ask questions."

"Sometimes the nurse will remind you of things you have been told."

"You will hears doors opening and closing throughout the test."

b. lights

"After the doctor takes pictures of the heart, he needs to turn out the lights. It won't be completely dark. During the test lights are turned on and off."

14. Describe the angiogram— at least one is done for all patients.

"In this test, medicine . . ." (avoid word dye) ". . . is put through the tube in your arm or groin; then many pictures are taken quickly. The clack-clack sounds you will hear are the pictures falling into a box. Children often wonder what is going on."

"The nurse will tell you when it's about to happen. During this time all the people in the room will step out into the hallway."

"You will know when the medicine is used because you will get a warm feeling in your chest which goes away quickly. It's supposed to feel like that. The special medicine allows the heart to show up on the film."

"After these pictures are taken, everyone comes back into the room."

15. Describe the Hydrogen Test. If a septal defect is suspected, anticipate that this test will be done.

"The nurse will hold a mask over your nose and mouth for a second to give you a puff of air. You will hear a sound like sh, sh."

16. Describe the end of the test—suturing and dressing.

"When the tests are over, the doctor removes the tube from your arm or groin. He may need to put little stitches in to close the opening. Maybe they won't be needed. Then he will place a bandage over the spot."

17. Tell child that he will be transported to another room for one last set of pictures before returning to his room.

This is done if K.U.B. x-rays are taken to determine any G.U. anomalies because medication is already present in the system.

18. Describe routine for child after he returns to unit:

    a. bed rest for 4 hours or longer
    b. force fluids to help get rid of medicine
    c. T., B.P.'s
    d. radial or pedal pulses
    e. regular dressing when vein has been used or pressure dressing when artery has been used

    End of session here. Resume after an interval.

19. Ask child simple questions to ascertain his understanding of the preceding material.

20. Tell child about preparation for test:

    a. tag on bed the night before the test

    "The NOTHING BY MOUTH tag means you won't be having anything to eat or drink after you go to bed; you won't have breakfast either. This is done to make sure your stomach will not be upset when you get medicines."

    b. transportation to catheterization room—he will be taken in his bed (If you are to accompany him, tell him so; if not, tell him that a nurse will be with him during the procedure.)

    c. pre-procedure medications. Demonstrate needle play and allow participation.

    "Before your test, we will give you medicines so that you will become sleepy and won't mind the long test (approximately 3 hours). You may want to sleep most of the time; it's all right to do so."

    This information is given at the end of the session. Otherwise, the child may

become excited so that previous information may not be heard.
See Needle Play, page 130.

21. Remind child that after the small needle prick to insert tube, he will not feel any hurt. Convey to child that whoever hurts him is sorry though they may not have time to tell him so.

22. Reassure child that no other part of the body will be tested or worked upon.

Use playful repetition to clarify operative site for child under 6. (See page 11.) Reassure older child directly.

23. Give permission to ask questions at any time and to discuss areas you might have missed, if any.

24. Play up rewards—that he will be able to talk to his family and friends about this exciting event; that he will see new things; he will meet many people.

This allows the memory of stressful procedures to be associated with bravery and the wish for good health.

25. Ascertain the child's understanding of your explanations by asking him simple questions in relation to body outline or doll and allowing him to attach ECG leads, restraints, catheter to doll.

Some children will not be able to verbalize answers to questions but may be able to draw responses on the body outline or to point to appropriate areas.

26. Delete Part 4; turn to Part 5.

Note: General anesthesia is used only in cases of severe aortic stenosis when a left ventricular puncture is necessary. In such a case, prepare the child for anesthesia. See Part 4.

PART 3. G

PREPARATION OF A CHILD FOR CARDIAC SURGERY
(Repair of Ventricular Septal Defect)

DIRECTIONS	COMMENTS AND EXAMPLES
1. Refer to Parts 1 and 2 before continuing.	
2. After determining the child's fantasy regarding illness and hospitalization, give him a simple explanation of the anatomy and physiology of the cardiac system. Introduce symptoms and attempt to relate them to his problem. Use a body outline for the child over 3½.	*For toddlers and Young 3's:* "The doctor is going to fix your heart." *Older 3's to 7 Group:* "The heart is in the middle of your chest. Its job is to send blood around the body taking food and nourishment to make you grow and stay strong. In your heart, you have a little hole that doesn't belong there. It makes more work for the heart. We don't know why; you were born that way. Your doctor knows how to sew up the hole so it will not cause you any trouble." *7 Years and Older:* Give same explanation as for older 3's to 7 group. In addition, use model and/or diagram of the heart.
3. If symptoms are absent, modify the approach.	"Although you haven't felt sick, we know that if your heart isn't fixed, it will give you trouble later on. We are going to take care of it now, so that you will continue to grow well."
4. Reassure the child that no one is to blame for his condition. Make it clear that neither his condition nor hospitalization is a punishment.	
5. Indicate operative site and postoperative appearance. a. incision	 "This is where the doctor will make an *opening* in your chest (either lateral or midline). Then he can sew up the hole in your heart." Draw incision on body outline or doll.

b. chest tube, sutures and bandage

"After your operation, there will be a tube coming from your chest to drain off old blood and air. The tube will be connected to a bag by the bedside. In about a day or so, the doctor will remove this tube because you won't need it any more. There will also be little black stitches that are used to close the opening. A large bandage on top will keep everything safe and clean."

c. pacemaker (if anticipated by catheterization data)

"You may find after the operation that a tiny wire has been placed under the skin where the doctor makes the opening. This wire is attached to a small box that looks like a pocket radio. It is used to regulate the heartbeat; to make sure that the heart beats as fast as it should. We won't be able to tell you now how long you will need this box, but we will let you know later." Show him a pacemaker.

d. Foley catheter (if used)

"The bladder is the place where urine (wee wee) stays. When the bladder is full you feel like urinating (making wee wee) and the urine comes out of the penis (or the little opening between the legs)." (Draw in bladder on outline.) "After the operation you will have a small tube going into the bladder to drain off the urine so that we know how much urine is made. This means that you *won't need to urinate.* Before long, this tube will come out and you will urinate just as you do now."

e. nasogastric tube (if used)

"When you wake up there will be a small tube going from your nose into your stomach (tummy). This will keep your stomach empty and it will also keep your stomach from being upset. It may be uncomfortable."

f. intravenous infusions, usually 2; one may be a cutdown

"Because you won't be able to eat for a while, you will have a tube going into your arm and leg. Through the tubes we can give you sugar water and medicines until you are allowed to eat again!"

g. ECG leads and monitors

"Do you remember having a picture of your heartbeat (electrocardiogram)?

When the operation is over, the doctor and nurses will want to watch your heartbeat for a while; so you will be wearing those metal plates and wires on your arms and legs. However instead of watching the heartbeat on a strip of paper, they will watch it on a TV screen, like this." Show patient a monitor.

h. endotracheal tube and Volume Control Respirator

"When you wake up, there will be a tube in your mouth to help you breathe deeply. The tube will be held in place by tape so that you won't be able to talk to us, but we will talk to you and you will hear us. If you want to tell us something, your nurse will give you pencil and paper to write notes." (Younger children may point to pictures.) "We know that having this tube in your throat will be uncomfortable, but you will be sleeping most of the first day and night. Usually the tube can be taken out the day after your operation."

6. Ask child simple questions to help him recall what you have told him and assist him in placing equipment on his doll (to visualize postoperative appearance) and to draw in responses on a body outline.

For complex surgery, the use of a doll is recommended, even for children over 7. Continue to use a body outline in conjunction with the doll for patients over 3½.

7. Reassure child that no other part of the body will be operated upon.

Use playful repetition to clarify operative area for the children under 6. (See page 11.) Reassure older child directly.

8. Introduce needle play related to blood work already experienced. Demonstrate and allow participation. See Needle Play, page 130.

This is introduced at the end of a session because it is quite exciting for the child. Preceding material may not be heard, otherwise.

9. Play up rewards. Tell the child that he will be able to talk to his family and friends about this exciting event—about the new

This allows the memory of stressful procedures to be associated with bravery and the wish for good health.

things he will see and do, and the people he will meet. Tell him that everyone will be surprised to hear about his hospitalization. Indicate that he will be able to show them how it was done on his patient doll.

10. Order Bennett or Bird respirator or blow bottles so that they will be available for the next teaching session.

End session here. Resume after an interval.

11. Ask the child simple questions to ascertain his understanding of the preceding material. Correct as necessary.

12. Introduce the croupette.

"About a day or 2 after the operation, the tube that helps you to breathe deeply will be taken out of your mouth. When this happens, your nurse will place a plastic tent over your bed or a plastic piece around your face. A vaporizer will pump cool air and moisture into the tent to help you breathe well and to make you more comfortable. The room will look misty (foggy)."

13. Introduce mistifier.

Show the child a croupette or face tent.

14. Introduce Bennett or Bird respirator or blow bottles.

"We will want you to breathe deeply and to cough up mucus (phlegm), like you do when you have a cold. This is hard to do all by yourself. So, we give you this breathing machine to help you do it. Sometimes your nurse will put medicine in here (nebulizer) to loosen the mucus so that you can cough it up more easily. This machine will be your friend; it will help you breathe deeply and get well faster."

Allow ample time for practice on respirator or bottles.

15. Introduce suctioning.

"Sometimes it is very difficult to get up the mucus (phlegm). This little tube goes down into the throat and pulls it up. It isn't so pleasant, but afterwards you will feel a lot better." Show him a suction machine or a model.

16. Explain turning and coughing. Demonstrate with patient. This is difficult for the child to learn, but staff in the Intensive Care Unit must have his cooperation.

"Because we know that it will be hard for you to cough after your operation, this is another way in which your nurse will help you. She will place a pillow on your chest or hold your chest with her hands, so that it won't hurt you so much."

Demonstrate this. Does the patient understand what is expected by:

1) take a deep breath
2) cough
3) cough up the mucus

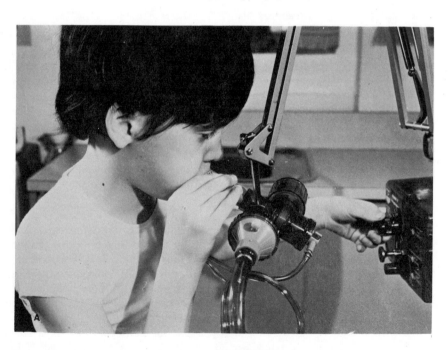

Fig. 6-4 A and B. When intricate and ominous equipment is introduced before it is actually needed, the child is more cooperative and less likely to become anxious. (photo 6-4 A by Steve Campus, photo 6-4 B by Hilary Smith)

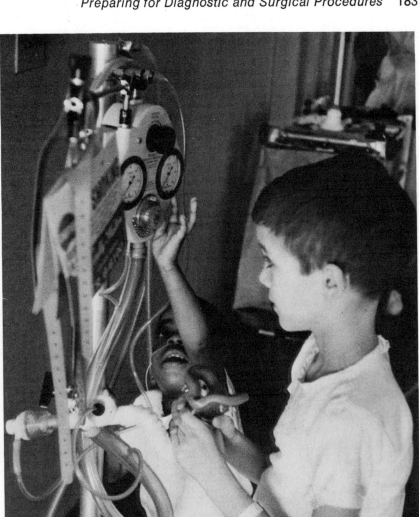

Figure 6-4 (*Continued*)

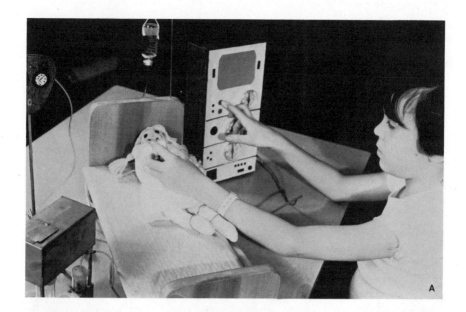

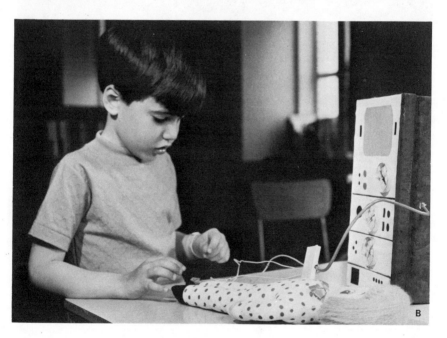

Fig. 6-5 A and B. The child learns that he will be required to cooperate with treatments that necessitate physical restraint and discomfort. Talking about how the puppets feel helps the child cope with the prolonged ordeal. (photos by Steve Campus)

17. Explain to the child that he will feel some pain (hurt) but that the nurses and doctors know how to take care of it with medicine.

"You may find it hard to keep from getting angry, but the nurses and doctors will appreciate cooperation. They know it isn't easy."

18. Explain that the room where he will be staying after the operation is usually a very noisy place; there is a great deal of activity and many people will visit him there, sometimes all at once.

19. Inform the child that he will be weighed daily on a stretcher scale (nude). Show him the scale if this is a routine.

Some children will resist getting onto the stretcher scale believing that they are going to the operating room again, if it is not explained in advance.

20. Place the child's teaching tools—doll, body outine, and other play materials— in a bag and secure to end of bed so that staff in the ICU will have these articles to help them care for the child.

21. Turn to Part 4.

PART 3. H
PREPARATION OF A CHILD FOR BRAIN SURGERY

DIRECTIONS	COMMENTS AND EXAMPLES

1. Refer to Parts 1 and 2 before continuing.

2. After determining the child's fantasy regarding hospitalization, illness, and his concept of the brain, give a simple explanation of the anatomy and physiology involved. Introduce symptoms and refer to diagnostic testing.

Because many children react unfavorably to discussion of treatment of the brain, it is advantageous to refer to the affected areas as nerve areas and inside the head.

Toddlers and Young 3's:

"The doctor knows how to make you feel better; to take away (whatever symptoms the child demonstrates). He is going to do an operation here . . ." (indicate on doll) ". . . to fix what is making you sick."

Older 3's to 7 Group

"You've had a great many tests lately (x-rays, pneumoencephalogram, electroencephalogram, spinal tap). By doing these tests, your doctor has found out what has been making you sick—why you have had movement of the eyes, difficulty walking and standing, speech problems or visual difficulty, headaches and vomiting" (whatever applies).

"The tests and the way you have been feeling tell your doctor that there is a small lump (growth) in your head that is pressing on some nerves (or a collection of fluid that is pressing on nerves). There are different kinds of nerves; some have to do with seeing, talking, hearing, smelling, swallowing. The growth he has found has been pressing on your _____ nerves. That's why your doctor has decided to do an operation to get rid of the growth (or fluid). This is where the operation is done, right here." Show on outline.

7 Years and Older:

A variation of the above. "As the growth gets larger it causes pressure and irritates the nerves that control sight, hearing, walking. Your problems tell us which nerves are affected. That's why your doctor has decided to remove the growth."

When symptoms are due to obstruction to the flow of cerebrospinal fluid—"The growth is blocking the movement of fluid that constantly flows around the brain and spinal cord." (Draw on outline.) "When this happens, pressure builds up and makes you feel uncomfortable and sick. That's why you have been irritable and tired, have been vomiting, have had difficulty with sight." (Say whatever applies.) "The doctor can remove the growth that is causing the blockage. That's why you are having the operation."

3. Explain area of incision and preparation of operative site.

For cerebral lesions the operative site is frontal behind the hairline; for cerebellar and brain stem lesions the incision is occipital.

"In order to do the operation, a part of your head needs to be shaved—just the section where the doctor makes the opening." (Children over 7 can be told that a bone wedge is removed so that the doctor can reach the affected part and that the bone is saved.) "After the hair grows in, the opening (incision) will no longer be noticeable. In the meantime, we can arrange your hair to cover the spot . . ." (if hair is long enough) ". . . or you may want to wear a scarf, wig, or cap."

4. Describe postoperative appearance and expectations:

   a. sutures

"When the operation is over the doctor closes the opening with black stitches, or the doctor replaces the bone to cover the spot so that it will be just as it was."

   b. bandage

"Then he winds a large bandage around your head. It will be very large and feel like a pillow for resting your head. It might look like a turban or helmet."

c. positioning of bed

"You might notice that your bed is turned around so that the head is at the foot. It will make it easier to take care of you this way."

d. positioning in bed and turning

"We will place you in bed according to the doctor's directions—flat and on your (unaffected) side—and we will turn you often."

e. suctioning

"Because it is quite hard to cough up mucus (phlegm) when you are flat in bed, we will help you do it. We have a little tube that goes down into the throat and pulls the mucus out. It's not too pleasant while it is being done. You might feel like gagging, but afterwards you will feel a lot better. It will help you breathe easier. Whoever does this knows how hard it is to bear and she is sorry there's no easier way." Show child a suction machine.

f. vital signs

"Your nurses will take your temperature, pulse and blood pressure very often. This is supposed to happen. These things tell us what needs to be done for you; for example, you may feel very warm, and we will need to make you feel cooler."

g. croupette or oxygen tent

"One of the ways we use to make you feel cooler is to place you in a plastic tent after the operation. A vaporizer will pump cool air and moisture into the tent. This is also used to help you breathe better and to make you more comfortable. I'll show you what the tent is like."

h. intravenous infusion

"For a while after the operation, you won't feel like eating or drinking. We know how to take care of you so that you will get the food and water you need to keep strong. The doctor places a tube in your vein (of arm or leg); it is connected to a bottle of sugar water. Your arm or leg will be placed on a small board to help you keep it from moving about."

i. elbow restraints and side rails

"Sometimes it is hard to remember not to touch the bandage on the head or to keep your arm still. If it is necessary, we will place loose ties around your arms and legs to help you remember." (Do not imply punishment.) "We will have side rails on your bed so that you will feel safe."

j. edema and discoloration (*In cases of frontal incision,* prepare the child and family for the likely possibility of head and facial edema —especially swelling of the eyelids—and discoloration around the eyes—ecchymoses.)

"Sometimes after this kind of operation there is swelling around the head, face and eyes. And the skin around the eyes may turn black and blue. This may not happen, but I'm telling you now so that you won't think it is unusual. If it does occur, it will disappear in a week or two. We can use ice around the face to make you feel more comfortable."

k. ventricular catheter

Explain the possibility of a ventricular catheter to the family. "Sometimes after surgery, a small tube (catheter) is placed within the brain for a few days to drain off excess fluid. This prevents the buildup of pressure. The fluid is collected in a bottle attached to the head of the bed. If it is used, you will see it right away. We don't know definitely now. We can tell your child postoperatively, if necessary."

l. tracheostomy (In cases of routine tracheostomy, prepare child in advance.)

In surgery involving the area of the brain stem, pressure on the respiratory center is anticipated. Some surgeons will routinely perform a tracheostomy. Tell the child and his family, "For this type of operation, we will do a procedure to make breathing easier. It is called a tracheostomy. A small opening is made into the windpipe (trachea). The opening can be seen on the neck. A tube will be inserted to keep the opening from blocking off. We will show you later how to hold your finger over the tube when you want to speak. If you forget to cover it, no sound will come out when you speak." Reintroduce suctioning.

5. Reassure child and family of the surgeon's and staff's skill in managing this type of problem; that it has been done many times.

This type of surgery is highly threatening to the child and family; they will need continuous support.

6. When a child appears stuporous or uncomprehending, caution family to refrain from discussing his condition in his presence. Direct them to explain activities and events as though he understands.

Frequently a child who is apparently comatose will comprehend what is said although he gives no clue.

7. Set up signals for the nonverbal child to indicate yes and no and to represent his needs. Inform staff and family of communication system.

8. Reassure child that no other part of the body will be operated upon.

Use playful repetition to clarify operative site for the child under 6. (See page 11.) Reassure older child directly.

9. Ask the child simple questions to ascertain his understanding of your teaching. Help him draw in answers on the body outline. Help young children attach equipment to a doll.

10. Play up rewards—how much he will have to tell his family and friends about the hospital, about the new things he has seen, and about the different people he has met.

This allows the memory of stressful procedures to be associated with bravery and the wish for good health.

11. Turn to Part 4. Before continuing, determine whether preoperative sedation is to be used. Central nervous system depressants are ordinarily eliminated before brain surgery.

Note: Because the performance of a ventriculogram requires the use of general anesthesia, surgery will follow directly when there is evidence of brain tumor. When surgery is dependent upon the results of this diagnostic procedure, the family and child must be prepared in advance.

PART 4.
GENERAL INSTRUCTIONS FOR ALL PATIENTS ON THE DAY BEFORE TREATMENT

DIRECTIONS	COMMENTS AND EXAMPLES
Explain imminent events to child.	
1. Fasting after bedtime and in the morning.	"You will find a tag on your bed that says NOTHING BY MOUTH. It means that after bedtime you will not be getting anything to eat or drink. You won't have any breakfast either; so, you may feel hungry and thirsty. We do this so that your stomach (tummy) will not be upset when we give you medicine before your operation."

If an intravenous feeding is anticipated, reintroduce it here. Explain that he will be fed again just as soon as he is able to tolerate it, and that he will be given fluids first. |
2. Explain pHisoHEX bath to make the skin very clean.	
3. Explain transportation to operating room in his own bed or on a stretcher. If you plan to accompany the child, tell him so.	This is one of the most supportive measures we can supply for the child. A familiar and supportive person who accompanies the child minimizes insecurity. When planned in advance, it can be managed.
Indicate to child that you know that children are usually lonely at these times and that they prefer their parents; but because parents can not go along, you will be there to be like his mother or father. Tell him parents will be waiting in his room (if true).	Try to bring along a favorite toy. Secure it to the bed.
4. Describe attire of anesthesia and operating room personnel.	"On the way, if you are not asleep, you'll probably see doctors and nurses in blue caps, masks and gowns. Did you ever see someone wearing a mask? Here they are

used to keep others from catching colds, if anyone has a cold."

Most young children associate masks with "bad guys" or games, so it is important to explain their use.

Give the child a disposable mask for play and to show his friends.

5. Explain anesthesia—that he will not be awake because he will be given a sweet smelling medicine by mask over the nose and mouth (modify for intravenous anesthesia); that he will not feel the operation nor remember it. Show him a mask and allow him to try it and handle it.

Many children show preoccupation with waking during the operation, or disbelief that they will not feel pain. Reassure child that there is a special doctor whose entire job is to see to it that the mask is kept in place and that everything goes well.

It is difficult to avoid the word "sleep" in describing anesthesia. Thus, it is important to differentiate between nighttime sleep and sleep induced by medication in order to avoid problems around bedtime later. Some children become fearful that other procedures will take place when they are asleep.

6. Introduce Recovery Room. Indicate that he will not return to his room directly but will go to the RR until he is fully awake. Explain that the people working there are trained especially to take care of patients who have just had operations. Indicate that the recovery room nurses will call his unit to let floor nurses know he has returned and that his nurse will come to see him right away (if true).

Describe attire of staff and the number of other patients there.

OR

7. Introduce Intensive Care Unit. Indicate that it is an area where the staff is trained to care for his kind of surgery or illness. Ex-

If the child is to go to an adult ICU, do not allow a visit preoperatively; it is much too threatening. If a child is to be sent to a pediatric ICU, arrange for him to visit in advance if you can determine ahead

plain the anticipated length of stay and that parents and staff will visit him there.

of time that it is not frightening. Otherwise, ask a member of the ICU staff to visit him in his own unit. Describe activities, noise and people of the ICU. Arrange for a member of the staff to accompany parents on their first visit to the ICU and to prepare them for child's appearance.

8. Discuss pain and its relief.

"After the operation, you may feel uncomfortable (feel some pain or hurt). The pain will mean that the operation is over and that the body is sore. We know how to take care of hurting with medicine. We usually know when you need it, or you can tell us when you need it."

9. Review information covered in Part 3. Ask simple questions to help child recall, in relation to body outline and doll. Evaluate how much has been retained. Repeat information as necessary. Encourage questions.

10. Explain preoperative medications that he will be receiving—that one (or 2) "shot" will make him drowsy and get him ready for the operation.

This aspect is covered at the end of the session because it is exciting for the child. We want to be assured of the child's attention to the preceding material.

Demonstrate needle play again and encourage participation. See Needle Play, page 130.

11. Turn to Part 5.

PART 5.
INSTRUCTIONS FOR ALL PATIENTS ON THE DAY OF SURGERY

DIRECTIONS	COMMENTS
1. Encourage parent or supportive adult to be present no matter how early surgery or procedure is scheduled.	Frequently parents believe that their presence is not important. They need to understand the child's point of view; i.e., that he needs his parents to help him cope with the stress to which he is exposed. Knowing that parents are waiting for him makes the whole event more bearable. It is reassuring for him to know that they are aware of what is happening to him.
	Parents need to know that even though adolescents may display an independent facade, they still have dependency needs which are intensified under stress.
	Despite the fact that young babies can not comprehend what is happening, they are able to pick up anxiety in others. As a result, they may appear irritable or restless. Pacifiers and rocking help to calm them.
	If parents are very anxious, just a brief visit to let the child know that they are there and will be waiting will suffice.
2. Review quickly the last minute events that are to take place. Tell child or parents that you believe that you have told them everything they need to know, but if there is anything that has not been explained, they should bring it up for discussion later.	
3. Prepare preoperative medications and place them out of sight in the child's room. When you are ready, tell him that it is time for his shots and proceed to administer medications *immediately*. Indicate that it will	A lapse of a few minutes is enough for the child to develop extreme anxiety. Once you have informed the child that it is time for injections, follow through quickly. There is no way to totally eliminate some discomfort—so the quicker the better.

hurt a bit; that it is unpleasant but has to be done. Do not ask child if it is all right to go ahead; he has no choice. Permit him to object or cry but direct him to hold still so that it can go faster. Tell him you have brought a helper with you to make it easier for him to hold still. Do not imply punishment.

Explain that the shots will make him sleepy, just as you told him they would. Allow quick needle play to help him master the situation. Young toddlers and babies respond well to cuddling.

A steady, calm voice communicates safety. Anything familiar is reassuring. Being friendly, scientific and chatty helps the older child during the procedure.

4. On call, accompany child to operating room. If he is awake, discuss with him the events taking place (include him in any conversations) and point out different personnel encountered.

5. Stay with child until he is anesthetized.

Most institutions will require the nurse or assigned staff member to change into appropriate clothing for this activity.

6. Turn to Part 6.

PART 6.

HELPING THE CHILD TO COPE WITH FEELINGS RELATED TO HOSPITALIZATION AND TREATMENT

Post-Procedural Period

DIRECTIONS	COMMENTS
1. Allow child to resume former activities as soon as possible, and to wear own clothing or hospital supplied daytime clothing.	Dressing and getting out of bed are immensely reassuring to the child. Even young babies and toddlers with I.V.'s can be picked up or positioned so that they may observe activities.
2. Allow opportunity for dramatic play. Have at child's disposal safe equipment which has been used in his treatment—stethoscope, tongue blades, blood pressure equipment; also doll, body outline and play materials representing equipment specific to his condition.	A hospital corner in the pediatric playroom provides an excellent opportunity for the expression of feelings and clarification of events.
3. For the verbal child, encourage talk about hospital experiences with staff, family, visitors and peers.	This can be done by merely asking the child what happened to him.
4. Encourage letter writing and telephoning as way of communicating with friends about experiences.	
5. Provide materials for child to draw or paint about hospital experience. Ask child to tell a story about his picture.	
6. Some children prefer to make a scrapbook with pictures cut out of medical or nursing journals. Ask child to write or tell a story related to them.	

7. Older children frequently prefer to keep diaries.

8. Encourage parents to photograph hospital scenes related to their child, so that he may have a picture history of events and can be reminded of his bravery.

The preceding measures give the child the opportunity to gain ego mastery of difficult situations by giving conscious thought to them. They provide also, the occasion for clarifying the difference between fantasy and reality; thus preventing the repression and retention of unrealistic fantasies.

9. Supply occupational and educational projects. Enroll in school and teen program if available.

Consult with school teacher, play and occupational therapists for suggestions.

10. Allow child to take home safe play materials. Interpret to parents the need to keep the subject of hospitalization and treatment open to discussion and clarification, in order that the experience can be integrated into the child's life.

This is especially true for the 3- to 6-year-olds, who need repeated assurance that they were in no way responsible for illness, as guilt is a major problem for this group (egocentric thinking).

11. Prepare parents for the kinds of behavior their child may demonstrate after discharge.

See Preparing Parents for Discharge of the Child, page 83.

12. Invite child to visit the unit after discharge, when he comes to clinic or the doctor's office. This provides the staff with an opportunity to evaluate the child's adjustment, and helps the child maintain contacts with staff. For children requiring frequent hospitalization, this facilitates future adjustment.

This revisitation helps to correct the distorted memories and diminishes anxiety in the event of future hospitalization.

PART 7.
BODY OUTLINES USED FOR CHILDREN AND PARENTS

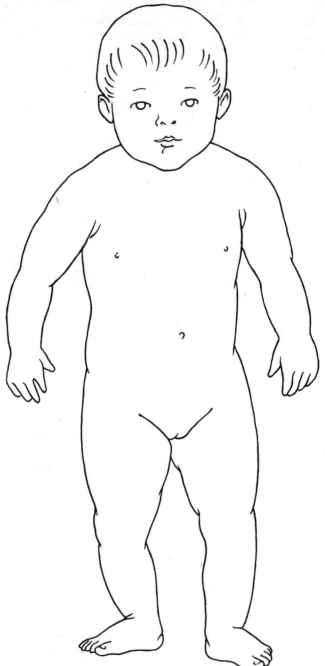

Fig. 6-6. (All body drawings by Melvin A. Miller)

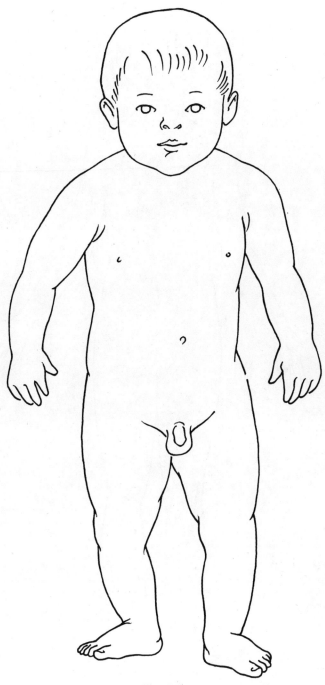

Fig. 6-7

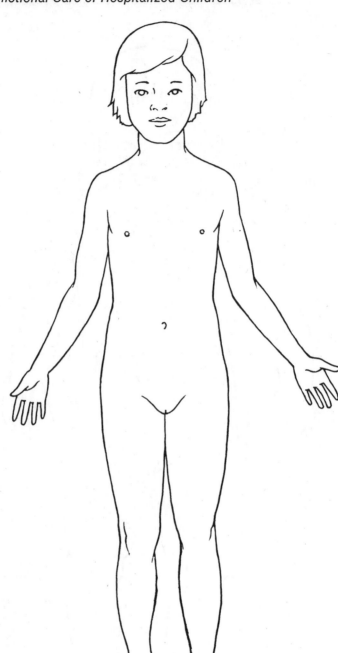

Fig. 6-8

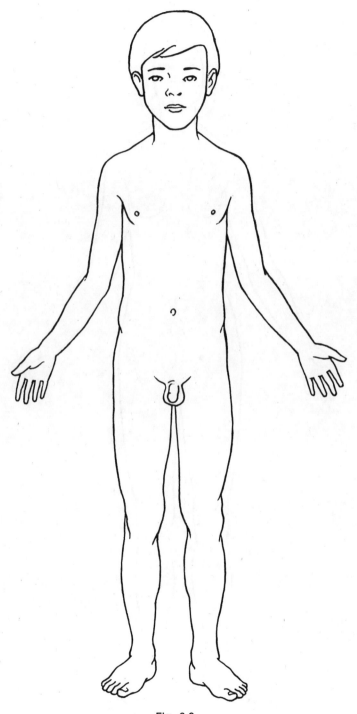

Fig. 6-9

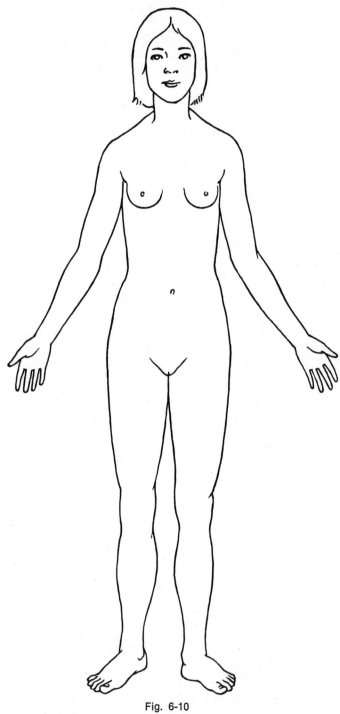

Fig. 6-10

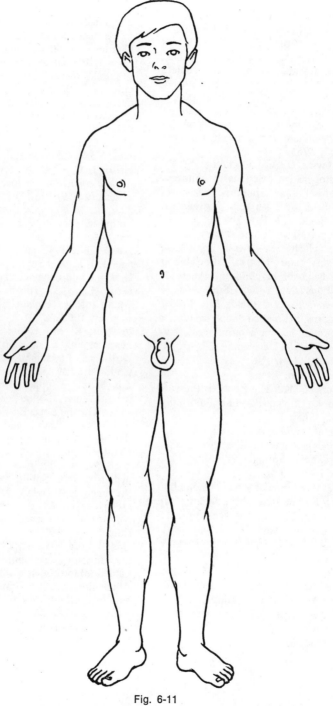

Fig. 6-11

BIBLIOGRAPHY

Brazelton, T. B., and Robey, J. S.: Observations of neonatal behavior. The effect of perinatal variables, in particular that of maternal medication. J. Amer. Acad. Child Psychiat., *4*:613, 1965.

Cassell, S.: The effect of brief puppet therapy upon the emotional resonses of children undergoing cardiac catheterization. J. Consult. Psychol., *29*:1, 1965.

Danilowicz, D. A., and Gabriel, H. P.: Postoperative reactions in children: "normal" and abnormal responses after cardiac surgery. Amer. J. Psychiat., *128*:185, 1971.

Davenport, H. T., and Werry, J. S.: The effect of general anesthesia, surgery and hospitalization upon the behavior of children. Amer. J. Orthopsychiat., *40*(5):806, 1970.

Donovan, E., and Gold, M.: Modal patterns in American adolescents. *In* Hoffman, L., and Hoffman, M.: Review of Child Development Research. vol. 2. New York, Russell Sage Foundation, 1966.

Escalona, S. K.: The Roots of Individuality. Chicago, Aldine Publishing Co., 1968.

Hammar, S. L., and Eddy, J. A.: Nursing Care of the Adolescent. New York, Springer Publishing Co., 1966.

Jessner, L.: Some observations on children hospitalized during latency. *In* Jessner, L., and Pavenstedt, E., (eds.): Dynamic Psychopathology in Childhood. New York, Grune & Stratton, 1959.

Josselyn, I. M.: Passivity. J. Amer. Acad. Child Psychiat., *7*:569, 1968.

Klaus, M. H., and Kennell, J. H.: Mothers separated from their newborn infants. Pediat. Clin. N. Amer., *17*:1015, 1970.

Levy, D. M.: The Demonstration Clinic: For the Psychological Study and Treatment of Mother and Child in Medical Practice. Springfield, Ill., Charles C Thomas, 1959.

Meeks, J. E.: Dispelling fears of the hospitalized child. Hospital Medicine, *6*:77, 1970.

Murphy, L. B.: Individualization of child care and its relation to environment. *In* Chandler, C., *et al.*: Early Child Care: The New Perspectives. New York, Atherton Press, 1968.

Richmond, J. B.: Child development: a basic science for pediatrics. Pediatrics, *39*:649, 1967.

Sander, L. W., *et al.*: Early mother-infant interaction and 24-hour patterns of activity and sleep. J. Amer. Acad. Child Psychiat., *9*:103, 1970.

Senn, M. J. E., and Solnit, A. J.: Problems in Child Behavior and Development. Chap. 3. The newborn and young infant. Philadelphia, Lea & Febiger, 1968.

Silberstein, R. M., *et al.*: Autoerotic head banging, a reflection on the opportunism of infants. J. Amer. Acad. Child Psychiat., *5*:235, 1966.

Smith, M.: Ego support for the child patient. Amer. J. Nurs., *63*:90, 1963.

Stechler, G., and Latz, E.: Some observations on attention and arousal in the human infant. J. Amer. Acad. Child Psychiat., *5*:517, 1966.

Wessel, M. A.: Training in neonatal pediatrics. *In* Solnit, A. J., and Provence, S. A. (eds.): Modern Perspectives in Child Development. New York, International Universities Press, 1963.

White, B., and Held, R.: Plasticity of sensorimotor development in the human infant. *In* Rosenblith, J., and Allinsmith, W.: The Causes of Behavior: Readings in Child Development and Educational Psychology. ed. 2. Rockleigh, N.J., Allyn & Bacon, 1966.

7

Loss, Grief and Death

THE PARENTS AND STAFF

Most people have similar grief reactions. Denial, protest, bewilderment, sadness, emptiness and idealization are seen in the early phase. Later on, with the slow acceptance of the reality of death, attachments are made stronger to existing relationships, and new relationships are sought. This is the hoped for outcome. However, many bereaved persons remain in one or another part of the early phase.

It is possible to anticipate a person's response to death. Almost everyone has some healthy resources for dealing with loss; usually a pattern has been already established. The shortest way to determine the pattern is to ask parents about recent separations, how the family as a group managed, to whom they turned during their troubles, and how they explained this illness to the other children.

The management of children and the family has been written about extensively. The need for privacy, sharing of grief, and empathy from the staff are obvious; however, allowance needs to be made for the work of the professionals to continue.

A systems approach* to a hospital floor is a concept that can be useful for effective planning. There needs to be at least a minimal capacity in personnel—medical and nursing students, doctors, nurses, social workers, orderlies, dietitians, elevator operators and parents—for dealing with loss. Although many routines continue, grieving people have a right to be protected from a "business-as-usual" atmosphere. All staff members can be respectful, conduct themselves with dignity, and remain available during the immediate bereavement.

A recurring problem is that of staff involvement. What is appropriate can be quite variable. Certainly, it is essential for the staff to be with the parents when they are told about the death. Although it may be painful,

---

* Systems theory states that for a large system to operate, there needs to be coordination among and smooth functioning within *all* subsystems.

the only way the staff can learn to cope with this kind of situation is for them to have experiences with it. Each professional team or floor should discuss in advance the procedures to be carried out, plan for this particular family, and make an assignment for one staff member to support the family after death. Thus, last minute confusion and unavailability can be avoided.

Contrariwise, overinvolvement and overavailability to the family causes the staff to have nonprofessional, social relationships with the family. This means that the staff becomes vulnerable to vicarious role playing and depressing identifications—they behave as a part of the family. If the staff becomes too emotionally involved with a family, they are unable to give support and may need it themselves. This violates the family's right to their own grief, calls attention to the staff's needs, and confuses roles; i.e., who is to console whom. Overfamiliarity with patients and families can only lead to difficulties. Furthermore, the staff, seeking protection from recurrent overinvolvement in grief reactions, may gradually come to withdraw from family involvements in an effort to prevent such entanglements.

The staff must be clear on what their professional role is. They need to determine the family's usual coping mechanisms that will tell how much support is needed and to whom the family will turn. In anticipation of death, the parents should be called in and the mourning process should be encouraged by talking about the dying child. The staff should join in the discussion with modesty in complimenting the parents on their handling of the illness; e.g., they should express the truth that in spite of more limited acquaintance with the child, they are deeply moved. In a kindly, practical manner the topic of how to tell the other siblings should be broached. (For recommendations in helping parents deal with siblings, see Chapter 4.)

Usually, the parents' guilt and repressed rage increases when their child has a long, terminal illness, or when there are repeated, near terminal episodes. In other words, recurring cycles of optimism and failure or the sight of an unremitting, hopeless process, expose parents to extreme psychic pain. The consequent upset might push the staff to offer the parents medications. Generally, the sedation of parents aborts the mourning process. Indications for this would be self-destructive acts, an impending psychosis, or the development of severe symptoms such as: prolonged insomnia, anorexia, severe withdrawal and panic. Psychiatric referral policies for these cases should be worked out in advance.

THE CHILD, PARENTS AND STAFF

Children will respond differently to death depending on their age; for example, children under 3 will fear separation from protecting and comforting adults (separation anxiety). They cannot comprehend the relationship of death to life until they develop a concept of infinite time.

The 3- to 6-year-old is more concerned with the illness as symbolic punishment for real or imagined wrongdoing. The child believes that the separation from parents that occurs with hospitalization is punishment for badness, and the painful procedures of tests and treatments augment this idea. Children may become depressed when these afflictions seem to be without an end point, because it implies that they will never be able to expiate their wrongdoings and regain the good graces of the adults they love.

Between the ages of 6 and 10, the child begins to fear death itself. This awareness is part of the general broadening of thinking that includes more realistic ideas of conception, family development, the contrast between animate and inanimate objects and a more worldly outlook. From this derives the idea that death is the cessation of life and of motion. Unlike sleep, its horrors are in unexpected pain, progressive mutilation and its mystery.

From the age of 10 on, a child can comprehend the permanence of death and its universality. The adolescent's response is similar to that of the adult although often sentimentalized. Also, it is at this time that youngsters are striving for achievements, success, independence, physical improvement and an ideal self-image. The child sees illness and possible death as impeding these goals. Thus, the child fears death-before-fulfillment: that the time and effort spent in growing up were wasted. Anxiety about death is particularly high in patients from future-oriented families, because they gain little solace from the past. Adolescents can become very depressed when faced with obvious body deterioration, dependency, and the loss of the social environment in which they have derived much pleasure and confidence from their age-specific skills.

Because at one time or another all medical persons will be asked by children who are going to die, "Am I going to die?", it is important to have in mind the reactions to death by different age levels, as well as some answers. Hesitation in answering, or awkwardness can only signal to the child one's own discomfort. There are general rules that the staff should follow when they discuss any delicate topic with children.

A plan needs to be made as follows: The parents should be consulted to determine their attitudes about death, how much information they are comfortable telling the child themselves, and how much they wish imparted by the staff. Next, information should be collected on what the child already knows or may suspect: (1) from what he has already been told; (2) from what the child has said; (3) from the way the child plays certain games; or (4) from the patients on the floor.

This rough picture of the child's orientation must be refined by turning the question around and asking the child directly what he knows about death and his own health status. The techniques for communication should be appropriate for the age so that a 4-year-old would be asked what happens to the toy dog when it is run over and killed by the toy car. On the other hand, the 9-year-old might talk about the terminal illness of one of the greats of baseball. The child deserves a response to any question. If a plan has not been made, it is best to say, "That's a good question; we will discuss it a little later." Then make a plan so the child will have an answer.

The most crucial determinant in answering or telling a child about death is how his parents feel about it. They too need to find some way to discuss death with their child. Often the parents are frightened and assume an attitude of deception. This can be corrosive because it alters relationships by severing the supportive intimacy all children need when they are stressed. Types of deception vary from the completely withdrawn or absent parent to the unfailingly cheery one, while some parents leave their tears unexplained. These parents have the idea that pretense with its insincerity, mystery, and maintenance of routine is better than a candid sharing of a mutual sadness; however, these maneuvers do not work. Unfortunately, most, if not all, children see through this pretense and develop fears that quite possibly are worse than the reality.

Furthermore, the hypocrisy of the parents degrades them and puts the child in the difficult position of the double bind; i.e., he is getting two messages—things are all right, and things are terrible—but is allowed to talk only about the first. In many instances, he anxiously refrains from telling what he knows in an effort to protect the parents! Thus, it is not surprising that the child will become increasingly docile, passive, and frightened the longer he is subjected to deception or silence. The parents' abdication leads to the child's withdrawal from reality. This has often been viewed by professionals as a calm and desirable occurrence. Nothing could be further from the truth because the child has been tragically left to face the future more alone than ever. With regression there is loss of identity. This is terrifying in that it causes a feeling of disintegrating functioning with attendant annihilation anxiety. A child who remains regressed is a treatment failure. For any age group, the loss of important people and loved ones is the paramount disaster.

The staff can help the parents be truthful with their child. The parents can tell him that they have deceived only in an attempt at wishful thinking (children do this all the time and understand the idea), and that their tears are partly from vexation with the illness that is keeping their loved one away from home and his usual activities. They can also tell their child that grown-ups like to show love with family activities (e.g., food, sports, and games); and that they have sad thoughts that he will not know how much they love him because they cannot do the usual family activities in the hospital.

The paths of honesty are not as variable as those of deception, for honesty about death leads directly to feelings of hopelessness, helplessness, and sadness. Honesty requires active skills to explore and integrate after the facts have been given, whereas deception is passive and conceals the facts leading to devious elaboration and subterfuge.

Honesty about death taxes the family and staff in the general areas of how well they cope with depression (hopelessness, helplessness, sadness), with death, with defeat of their powers to nurture their child, and with treatment that might lead to anger and humiliation. As a guideline, an attitude of "making-the-best-of-a-bad-deal" and making the most of the time remaining seem to be effective with those children and adults who cannot be comforted by religious beliefs. Heroic efforts such as Gunther's *Death Be Not Proud,* Hersey's *The Wall,* and *Anne Frank: The Diary of a Young Girl* illustrate the kinds of achievements that can occur as a result of challenge to life and relationships. It is always a surprise to adults, who have a romantic view of childhood, that children have the capacity to comprehend a "making-the-best-of-it" attitude and are in some ways inventive and practical about their afflictions. However, their inventiveness and play of mind to develop new solutions depends on keeping their anxiety at a minimum.

The first anxiety concerns immediacy—to know that death is not in the near future is reassuring. On the other hand, when to tell a child he is not going to recover requires the most profound clinical judgment based on a truly caring hospital environment. The danger of too early disclosure (as in the case of leukemia) burdens the child and parents and disrupts normal relationships. Too late disclosure leaves the child to grapple with this knowledge in solitude. He inevitably knows the truth (see Waechter).[1] Thus the issues are how and when to facilitate a child's discussing death, rather than should there be such a dialogue.

Not to be omitted is the staff and parental resistance that expresses itself in distorting the above ideas. There may be irrational fears that the mental health team recommends all terminal children be told, indiscriminately, that they are going to die. If this develops, it means that the staff and parents need more education and support.

The anxieties of each age are noted above; therefore, it follows that the constancy and physical closeness of parents is most important to the child under 3. In general, the more a child experiences constancy and continuity with parents, the less anxiety he will suffer. For the 3- to 6-year-old, closeness retains its helpfulness, but talking about illness—that it is not related to bad actions, that love is not contingent on certain behavior—will decrease anxiety. Constancy is based on maintaining limit setting and discipline, too.

From 6 on, the child is comforted if he is given details of what is to come with assurances that there will be little or no pain, that surprises will be kept to a minimum, and that alternative skills can be developed for other academic and athletic distinctions. To allay anxiety of the adolescent requires more emphasis on present achievements, continuity of peer relationships, de-emphasis on physical perfection, development of the mind, learning to enjoy memory and perhaps altruistic assistance to the grown-ups who find death unbearable.

There is a special category of the problem: the child who is kept alive by artificial, mechanical means. Parents may at first give approval to keep their child alive in this way, but later become regretful. When they request the life-sustaining treatment be stopped, the staff should consider this request in the larger context of how the family may be suffering and depleted, emotionally and financially. There needs to be a departmental policy for this contingency.

Parental guilt may be somewhat alleviated by transferring responsibility for the decision to the impersonal, inevitable disease process. The parents should know that the idea of untreatability is based upon scientific diagnosis and probability, not on the parents' emotional exhaustion.

Lastly, parents need follow-up to assay residual effects on them and on young members of the family. Staff and private pediatricians can encourage parents to make return visits in order to discuss how the family has adapted. A covering-over process is looked for whereby healthy life skills and defenses continue and the loved one is remembered with warmth. On the other hand, the physician should cautiously explore the reaction to the recent loss if parents and siblings show signs of: unresolved depression, yearnings for sickness, morbid preoccupations, and poor performance at work or school. Psychiatric evaluation is indicated when reactions appear intense or chronic.

DEATH AND CHILDHOOD*

	BEFORE		DURING			AFTER		
Child	*Ideas on Death*	*Death & Stage Anxieties*	*Sudden*	*Acute*	*Chronic*	*Sudden*	*Acute*	*Chronic*
0–5	abandonment punishment	fear of loss of love		avoidance of pain need for love guilt (bad) regression denial	withdrawal separation anxiety guilt (religious) regression denial			
5–10	concepts of inevitability confusion	castration anxiety						
10–15	reality	control of body and other developmental tasks		depression despair for future	depression despair anxiety anger			
Parents	*Sudden*	*Acute* — anxiety concern hopefulness	*Chronic* — premature mourning anticipatory grief, guilt, reaction formation and displacements, need for information	desperate concern denial guilt	denial remorse resurgence of love	guilt mourning	anger at M.D. need for follow-up over-idealizing fantasy loss	remorse relief and guilt
			disbelief displaced rage accelerated grief prolonged numbness					
Siblings								
0–5	reactions to changes in parents (sense of loss of love and withdrawal)						1. respond to reaction of parents	
5–10	concern re their implication fearful for themselves						2. survivor guilt	
10–15	generally supportive							
Staff	anxiety conspiracy of silence		reaction: withdrawal tasks: 1. correct distortions, e.g., "am I safe?"; "will someone be with me?"; "will I be helped to feel better?" 2. comfort parents 3. allow hope and promote feeling of actively coping 4. protect dignity of patient				need for after care of survivors autopsy request tact accurate information regarding disposal of body delay billing	

* From Lewis, M.: Clinical Aspects of Child Development. P. 198. Philadelphia, Lea & Febiger, 1971.

REFERENCE

1. Blake, F., Wright, F., and Waechter, E.: Nursing Care of Children. ed. 8, pp. 42-43. Philadelphia, J. B. Lippincott, 1970. (*See also* Waechter, E.: Death Anxiety in Children with Fatal Illness. Unpublished Doctoral Dissertation. Stanford University, 1968.)

BIBLIOGRAPHY

Hamovitch, M. B.: The Parent and the Fatally Ill Child. Los Angeles, Delmar Publishing Co., 1964.

Kennell, J. H., Slyter, H., and Klaus, M. H.: The mourning response of parents to the death of a newborn infant. New Eng. J. Med., 283:344, 1970.

Kubler-Ross, E.: On Death and Dying. New York, Macmillan, 1970.

Lindemann, E.: Symptomatology and management of acute grief. Amer. J. Psychiat., 101:141, 1944.

Rochlin, G.: Griefs and Discontents: The Forces of Change. Boston, Little, Brown & Co., 1965.

Solnit, A. J., and Green, A.: The pediatric management of the dying child, Part II: The child's reaction to the fear of dying. *In* Solnit, A. J., and Provence, S. A. (eds.): Modern Perspectives in Child Development. New York, International Universities Press, 1963.

Wiener, J. M.: Response of medical personnel to the fatal illness of a child. *In* Schoenberg, B. *et al.* (eds.): Loss and Grief: Psychological Management in Medical Practice. New York, Columbia University Press, 1970.

8

The Mental Health Team in Action

The following case summaries are only a small selection from the approximately 500 children who come to the attention of the mental health team yearly. This chapter is a sampling of typical adaptational difficulties. Each case illustrates environmental approaches and background skills described in the other chapters. The dramatic, immediate results in many children were usual and a major factor in gathering support for this program from new staff. The lack of complication in the case descriptions is partly in the interest of clear exposition. In fact, as often as not, a treatment plan was arrived at through negotiation and compromise. This then had to be implemented against the resistance of those who were outwardly compromising to the plan but still had degrees of subtle emotional opposition. Open disagreement was always more productive, because it allowed clarification and healthy debate. This often led to an arrangement in which a trial change of environment taught everyone the most effective approach.

ANTHONY – EIGHT MONTHS

Failed to Thrive

Mrs. C. was concerned because Anthony was not growing as well as her 3 older children. He was not hearty, did not eat as well, vomited easily, and did not respond happily to his environment. In effect, his mother derived little pleasure from caring for him.

One look confirmed Mrs. C.'s description. Anthony appeared to be suffering from a nutritional or malabsorption problem. Thorough diagnostic work was performed but the results were negative.

The possibility of inadequate sensory and tactile stimulation was considered. Thereafter, Anthony was bombarded with stimuli—music, singing, rocking, cuddling and much activity—but nothing about him changed. This circus atmosphere came to an abrupt stop one afternoon after several members of the staff witnessed Anthony and his mother together. They discovered that his mother also believed in highly stimulating interactions; she petted, stroked, shook and jostled him without mercy until he vomited. On this occasion his vomitus was bright red. Panicked, Mrs. C. rushed him into the hallway screaming for help. Anthony screamed too.

The chaos diminished when one of the nurses casually reported that he had eaten beets for lunch. It took a while to calm Mrs. C. who kept expressing concern that the staff would blame her for doing something wrong.

It was a valuable experience. This convinced the staff that it was not a case of understimulation—just the wrong stimulation. A detailed account of Anthony's daily home routine confirmed this. He was fed in front of a television set, in the company of 3 young children who were all competing for the attention of their harassed mother.

We succeeded in gaining Mrs. C's cooperation in trying a different approach in the hospital environmental. Anthony was:

1. Placed in the quiet infants' room.

2. Assigned to one nurse and his mother who gave him one feeding daily with the support and supervision of the nurse assigned. Mrs. C was assured that her mothering techniques were very good but that some babies were more sensitive and needed more subtle management.

3. Received quiet stimulation such as rocking, soft music, gentle handling, subdued lighting and bright mobiles. His nurse was directed to repeat his vocalizations as a method of rewarding and encouraging him.

The results were dramatic. Anthony settled down to a routine quickly. He stopped vomiting, gained weight and smiled readily. Without any persuasion, his mother decided that she could find a quiet place to feed the baby at home as well as provide activities for the others at the same time. She was grateful to be assured that she was a good mother.

After his discharge, Anthony was followed in the outpatient department. He continued to thrive and developed into a robust boy from whom his mother derived much satisfaction.

CALTON – EIGHT MONTHS
Ruminated

Calton was admitted because of low body weight and rumination (chewing and gargling of partly digested food and a dribbling form of vomiting). The usual vigorous hospital diagnostic work-up proved negative.

A conference was held to pool the knowledge everyone had about this baby. The nurses had learned that throughout this child's first months of life, he had been sleeping in a succession of temporary locations and was handled and fed according to the mother's schedule as an amateur entertainer. A chance remark that his mother made to a staff member indicated that she resented this child who was interfering with her career. Also the staff reported that Calton was unable to maintain eye contact, arched his back and became stiff when held, moved his fingers in front of his face, and rolled his head from side to side. A tentative conclusion was that this child was suffering from maternal deprivation. One nurse on each shift was assigned to care for him, and interfering contacts were kept to a minimum. His nurses were directed to respond to his crying immediately and to ignore the rumination. In this way, crying was reinforced as a more satisfactory way of getting attention and showing distress. Within 12 days the rumination diminished and Calton was able to maintain eye contact for several seconds.

Because the vomiting did not stop completely and because weight gain was minimal, the medical staff decided to reinstitute further vigorous diagnostic testing to account for calories that were being swallowed but not reflected on the scale. The rumination returned in full force, and eye contact stopped with a change in the nursing assignments. The staff became anxious as the child slowly continued to lose weight despite the introduction of nasogastric tube feedings.

Another conference was held at which time the staff disagreed over the validity of the small improvement made initially, and on the feeding techniques to ensure adequate nutrition. With reluctance and amid the rumor that the psychiatrist's recommendation of low stimulation actually meant an isolation room, a maternal regimen was finally reinstituted. Calton was placed in a quiet room, assigned one nurse per shift, and protected against sudden changes of light and noise.

It took several days for the infant to begin to thrive. Before long however, he gained significant weight, became more sociable, and ruminated rarely. Over a period of several weeks he began to sit, crawl, and progress developmentally. Eventually, he was ready for foster family placement. The follow-up was uneventful.

At a later staff conference, the management of Calton and others with similar symptoms was reviewed in the light of growing literature on the failure-to-thrive syndrome. As a result the doctors were willing to accept a less rigid approach to the treatment of these children. A meeting was planned at the departmental level to establish policy in these cases because bias prevented an individualized approach.

PHILIP – AGE TWO-AND-A-HALF

Resumed Growth—Physical, Emotional and Intellectual —During Hospitalization

Despite his hearty eating, Philip's mother noted that he had ceased to grow after the age of 1½ years. He was admitted for diagnostic testing and observation that required long-term hospitalization. Separation from his family appeared to pose no problem for this toddler; he was immediately at home and courted relationships with all members of the staff indiscriminately.

A charmer, before long he had everyone vying for his attention. He was able to manipulate people into giving him extra treats and privileges forbidden to the other children. Whenever he was refused a request, he found personnel from other floors to do his bidding. He had a following from every department connected with his unit. His maneuvers were so successful that it became obvious that he was completely undisciplined. His tantrums were catered to and there were no limits placed on his behavior.

At first Philip seemed excessively concerned with cleanliness. He became upset if his clothes and hands were soiled; he was rigid in his eating habits and became anxious whenever he dropped or touched food. He wanted everything cleaned up at once.

Philip became the subject of a nursing conference because of the premature versatility of his relationships, his overconcern with cleanliness, and because his parents were not visiting regularly. The following plan was put into operation:

1. Assign one nurse as chief mother substitute and another staff member to relieve her. Others are to resist involvement with Philip and to direct him to his mother substitutes for gratification.

2. Disregard tantrums and do not reinforce this behavior by giving in to it.

3. Send Philip to the playroom regularly and introduce him to finger painting, play dough, soap and water play.

4. Mother substitutes are to (a) encourage autonomy by preserving the skills already mastered—toilet training, dressing, feeding himself without help; (b) play games, sing and read to him, teach him rhymes and new words; (c) allow dramatic play related to procedures experienced, especially needle play.

5. Encourage parents to visit regularly, to leave family photos and to allow Philip to telephone home daily.

6. Ask for a social service intervention to determine home situation and to counsel mother.

7. Observe Philip's relationship to his parents during visiting periods.

At first, both Philip and the staff balked at the curtailment in his relationships; it was gratifying for some personnel to be Philip's rescuers. The restriction for Philip meant the curbing of his manipulative power. It took constant vigilance initially to ensure adherence to the plan. Before long, Philip learned that his needs were supplied by 2 people. As his relationships were strengthened with them, he naturally preferred them to others. After these relationships developed, it was easy to set limits on his behavior, because disapproval from his special nurses was now meaningful to him.

Philip's first experience with play dough and water caused him some difficulty. He frequently looked to those around him for their reactions. Once convinced that the staff would not be punitive, he derived great pleasure from these activities. He showed less concern about soiling, often eating with his hands, and once he was seen playing with feces.

With encouragement and praise, Philip maintained his former skills. In addition, he showed much curiosity, learned games and songs, and increased his vocabulary rapidly. He enjoyed playing doctor on his patient doll and displayed understanding of the procedures. Thus, his tantrums subsided when avenues for expression were provided.

It was difficult to persuade Philip's mother to visit because she had no one to care for her other children. Furthermore, she did not enjoy visiting because Philip refused to go to her voluntarily. Every time she visited, she disapproved of his disheveled appearance and would wash his hands and rearrange his clothes. She believed that the staff had spoiled him and it took some effort to convince her that we did not intend to usurp her maternal role. We explained that Philip's reaction to her was his way of expressing his anger at not having seen her for a long time. She agreed to call daily and to accept social service help.

During the latter part of his hospitalization, Philip began to gain weight. In order to ensure his progress, the staff arranged close social service follow-up with tentative plans for foster home placement if counseling of parents was not influential in his being more welcome at home.

NICOLAS – AGE THREE

Refused to Sleep in his Room

The night staff reported that Nicky had not slept for 6 nights. He cried to be let out of his room: sometimes he called for his mother. Medication was not effective in promoting sleep. On a few occasions he was taken into the dayroom where he promptly fell asleep on a chair or sofa. During the day, Nicky was groggy and liked to curl up for catnaps in any area other than his own unit. It was difficult to keep him in his room except when his family was present. Most of the time, he closed the door and remained outside, directing everyone else to do the same.

This behavior began the night following surgery for hypospadias repair. His mother believed that it was due to separation anxiety; Nicky was obviously calmer and more cooperative in her presence. This possibility was considered, but it did not account for his sleeping at night when the location was changed. This led to the supposition that Nicky's difficulty probably was related to an association between sleeping in bed and going to the operating room. He had received preoperative medications in his room and was transported to surgery in bed.

We decided to observe Nicky's play in the miniature hospital. The plan was to use the miniature hospital as a diagnostic tool to externalize the child's problem; to use dramatic play as a therapeutic tool as a way of relieving tensions and setting the boundaries between reality and fantasy.

In the first session he vacated all patient dolls and furniture from the bedroom areas; he then placed the patient dolls in the nurses' station, the toy chest, and outside of the hospital area. When asked what the dolls were doing in these places, he said that they were asleep. When he was asked, "Why there?", he said it was better that way. We asked him what happened to the boys and girls when they remained in their own rooms. He said that fires happened there and then he labeled the anesthesia and treatment rooms as fire areas too.

This episode made it possible for us to point out to him, over and over again, where the fire rooms were (anesthesia and treatment rooms). We explained that fires did not happen in the bedrooms and that it was safe to sleep there. Also, we made the distinction between nighttime sleep and drug-induced sleep. Nicky ended his play abruptly stating that he did not like to play because it made fires. When asked where the fires were, he clutched his penis.

The staff and his mother, who was an eager participant, were directed to reinforce the explanations made during the day. There was no change in Nicky's behavior after the first session. However, he was keen on playing in the model hospital again. During the second session, essentially the same themes prevailed; i.e., removing beds and dolls from the "boo-boo" rooms. On this occasion he was asked what brought little boys to the hospital. He had a quick answer, "because they make do do in their pants and touch their pee pees." Therefore, as previously, the staff took the opportunity to clarify reality for him. This time the session ended differently. Before he left the playroom Nicky returned the dolls and beds to the bedroom areas. Thereafter, his sleep problem disappeared and we knew that he understood our explanations.

However, we did have reason for concern later. Just before discharge it was decided that Nicky needed to have deep sutures removed under anesthesia. Precautions were taken in order to prevent a recurrence of the old problem. This time he was given medication in the treatment room, and he was transported to the operating room on a stretcher. This procedure proved to be a good move because there was no more difficulty.

Because of egocentric thinking at this age, the relief Nicky experienced would only be temporary. His parents were encouraged to reinforce reality by keeping the subject of hospitalization and treatment open for discussion and by assuring him that he was not responsible for his condition.

JACK — AGE FOUR

Suffered Acute Depression

Jack was originally admitted for repair of a chest deformity. He acquired a staphylococcus infection postoperatively. As a result, he was placed in isolation for 2 weeks and received medication intramuscularly every 6 hours.

Following the period of isolation, severe depression brought him to the attention of the mental health consultant. It was reported that Jack had not been prepared for hospitalization. His parents appeared overwhelmed by the experience and attempted to keep information from their child for his protection. Jack's response was to withdraw from all activity, shun the company of his parents and staff, and vomit repeatedly when forcibly fed by his parents.

On the basis of the information brought out in a staff conference, the following plan was initiated:

1. Assign nursing personnel to him consistently.

2. Ascertain Jack's understanding of his hospitalization and treatment and clarify misconceptions; to communicate with him by the use of drawings and encourage the expression of feelings by play acting treatments on his teddy bear.

3. Deal with separation anxiety by (a) encouraging his parents to visit consistently; (b) allowing Jack to telephone his family daily; (c) asking

parents to bring in family photos and (d) talking to him in terms of when he is home again.

4. Interpret to parents the necessity for giving explanations to children and of visiting regularly in order to maintain the child's trust.

5. Gain parents' cooperation in managing the eating problem by de-emphasizing it.

Initially Jack talked to no one; thus, it was not possible to elicit his understanding of what had happened to him. Instead, his nurse explained to the teddy bear, who had the role of the patient, the nature of the surgery and the kinds of routines and procedures that Jack had personally experienced. She gave teddy his first injection and had the bear object loudly and demand a proper explanation for the painful needle. Following this, Jack gave injections too but remained silent until he received his next intramuscular injection. His first expression to the nurse was, "Now you're really getting me mad."

Safe equipment such as syringes without needles, bandages, and adhesives were left at his bedside for leisurely play. On one occasion he taped the bear to the bedside and explained that teddy was being punished for not eating. When he was asked what kept him from eating, Jack replied, "Teddy won't eat because he feels choked."

Before long, Jack was telling us how much he missed his mother, although he continued to ignore her presence when she visited. His mother believed that he did not need her and decided to stop visiting altogether. When she explained this feeling to Jack's nurse, the latter took the opportunity to interpret his behavior. She explained that Jack's behavior was his way of retaliating for what he perceived to be his mother's abandonment of him (in fact, it is not unusual for young children to react in this manner). It was made clear to her that he asked for her frequently and that no one could adequately substitute for her.

As a result of the discussion, a regular visiting pattern was established and other measures to lessen the mother's separation anxiety were carried out. The parents were included in Jack's teaching and were encouraged to reinforce it. Also they agreed to avoid being present at mealtime, because they believed that they could not refrain from force feeding.

Within 2 days, Jack's vomiting stopped, even during times when his parents coaxed him to eat (other than mealtime). He began to relate to other children and was able to object verbally to what he considered "choking" treatment.

The staff was delighted with his behavior and did not anticipate that Jack's parents would be less so. Apparently, his parents did not consider an outgoing, expressive child to be an asset. At a staff conference, we discussed the reasons for the parents' hostile attitude to what we termed Jack's improvement. We had assumed that Jack's former behavior was a problem to his parents, when in actuality, it was not. In retrospect, no one could recall the parents voicing any concern. We agreed that there had not been enough work done with the parents to explore their ideas and feelings regarding the events taking place. We had not adequately considered the mother's belief that Jack did not need her anymore. To her it probably meant that she had no more function and that the staff could do better.

The best recommendation for this kind of problem is psychiatric evaluation of the mother. Had our relationship with this family been better, this might have been possible. Under the circumstances, however, we could not expect Jack's behavior at discharge to be long-lived.

ROBINSON — AGE FIVE

Acted Out His Castration Fantasy

Uncircumcised in infancy, Robbie, age 5, was admitted for elective surgery to correct the situation at his father's request.

Robbie was told that the procedure involved the removal of foreskin, that his penis would be sore afterwards but that it would all be there. Nevertheless, he was not a willing candidate; preoperatively, he was uncooperative and hyperactive.

Postoperatively, Robbie was agitated and cried a great deal. He was observed on several occasions sitting on the edge of a chair in the hallway, pulling up his gown to expose his genitalia as different staff members passed. Each time he was told that his penis looked sore but that it was all there and that before long he would notice that it looked better too. At first he was encouraged to repair broken toys (restitutive play) and then to use syringes and water pistols to play out the pleasure in the function of the penis. He appeared to progress well on this regimen and the staff was greatly relieved. By chance, however, just prior to his discharge, Robbie was examining his penis at his bedside as a woman visitor approached him. She reacted hysterically—screaming for a nurse to come see what had happened to the poor child. Robbie's reaction was even more intense. He began to howl like a wounded animal and was inconsolable. Not long afterwards, he was found wearing a girl's dress. He was assured over and over again that his penis was intact and that he was still a boy. The staff was unanimous in recommending further treatment. He was referred to Child Psychiatry on an outpatient basis.

Although this child's reaction was more prolonged and intense than usual, it is not atypical for children between the ages of 3 to 6, since preoccupation with mutilation and castration is prominent. Ideally, the stage of emotional development is one of the criteria considered in the selection of patients for elective surgery. The staff can assume that regardless of age, however, a child will have castration fears from procedures involving the genitals.

In Robbie's case, he was predisposed to difficulty. At a vulnerable period, he was to have surgery on a highly symbolized area of his body and for no apparent flaw. The parents' motivation for having Robbie circumcised at this particular time and other factors that predisposed him to a major disturbance were unclear.

The plan for managing this child involved (a) a thorough explanation of the surgery and related events, (b) repeated clarification of reality that his penis was intact), (c) use of restitutive play, and (d) psychiatric follow-up.

ALEX – AGE FIVE

Showed Bereavement and Feelings of Guilt

Alex was a 5-year-old boy whose mother died 3 months before he was admitted for the correction of a congenitally deformed penis (hypospadias). He clung to all the nurses that came by his bed, cried, and whimpered continuously. Despite this, the entire staff found him likeable and was sympathetic to him. He spoke about his mother and of how he missed her to one intern in particular. However, his talk was illogical, and he often stopped in the middle of a sentence or changed the subject.

At a staff conference, it was decided that a boy of this age, who had already had 2 stressful experiences (loss of mother and surgery), would tend to view these experiences as being related. They believed he needed to talk about his ideas of how his mother died, whether her death was caused by anything he had done, and whether the hospitalization and surgery were evidence of his badness and were punishment for his mother's death and his other wrongdoings. One person was assigned to Alex to talk with him and play out his ideas: on his own mortality and that his mother might not have left him if he had been a more lovable person.

Unfortunately, Alex was discharged before the plan could be carried out. On a return visit to the surgical follow-up clinic, it was noted that

Alex was depressed, more taciturn, and unwilling to attend school. At this time, the mental health nurse went over most of the issues that had been discussed at the conference. Alex became almost instantly loquacious and happier in his mood. His aunt was informed of the conference and was told to reinforce Alex's confidence by telling him whenever the opportunity arose how much his mother loved him, doing wrong does not result in horrible consequences, it is unlikely for him to die, and that his mother would be proud of his ability to talk about his worries. He was given a photo of his mother to carry with him and a hospital card with the names of staff he could visit in the coming months.

RUTH – AGE FIVE

Developed Nightmares After Cardiac Surgery

Ruth was a cooperative, docile child. She participated in the elaborate preparations indicated for major cardiac surgery and appeared to tolerate the stress remarkably well.

Postoperatively, Ruth's difficulties did not become apparent until she was returned to her own room after 48 hours in the Intensive Care Unit. Her mother, who stayed with her continuously, reported that Ruth was having such frightful nightmares that she was trying to avoid sleep altogether. The usual reassurances of telling her that the dreams were not real, of leaving a light on, and of having her mother close by did not help. Medication for sleep was tried without success.

During the day, Ruth was irritable, clinging and uncooperative. Her mother was alarmed and asked for direction.

There was no doubt that Ruth was reacting to the ordeal that she had undergone and was attempting to work out her experiences during sleep. The objective was to help her master the problem in her waking hours. Our routine practice of helping children to cope with hospitalization by allowing them to reenact experiences in dramatic play was completely rejected by Ruth. She refused contact with her preoperative doll on which she had practiced so compliantly those procedures she herself would undergo. It was too direct an approach for her. Instead, the staff used a method that Ruth found tolerable and that also employed her mother's artistic talents.

We avoided talk and play that concerned Ruth directly. Instead, we focused attention on a fictitious character named Evelyn, who was to be admitted to the pediatric department for chest surgery. Ruth and her mother occupied themselves with preparing a booklet on the kinds of things Evelyn needed to know—the people she would meet, the procedures she would undergo, and the fun activities in which she would participate. In addition, other patients on the unit were singled out as having similar or different experiences as Evelyn and their reactions were discussed openly. Eventually it was possible for Ruth to identify with Evelyn and to talk about herself and Evelyn interchangeably. When this occurred, she had no difficulty in playing with her own doll—inserting and removing chest tubes, I.V.'s, bandages and giving countless injections—with appropriate affect, sometimes in the role of doctor or nurse and at other times as the victim. Within 2 days, the nightmares disappeared. Convalescence proceeded satisfactorily. Her mother was encouraged to continue the play activities after discharge.

The plan for this child focused on helping her to cope with traumatic experiences by bringing them into conscious awareness. This involved (a) recalling the events and lessening her anxiety by using indirect methods (i.e., substituting a fictitious character and other children as the subjects); (b) turning passive experiences into active ones in order to master them and giving alternative meanings to real events; (c) using her mother, the most trusted person in her life as the therapist; and, (d) encouraging expression of feelings and enacting events through play after hospitalization.

VALERIE — AGE FIVE

Was A Champion Manipulator

Although Val came to us with a variety of behavior problems, in addition to chronic kidney disease, nothing about her provoked so much response from hospital personnel as did her refusal to eat at mealtime. In short order, she managed to win the attention of people from many different departments—physicians, nurses, dietitians, cleaning and laundry personnel, and ever changing visitors. She was so appealing—cute, little, sick and abandoned by her mother. Everyone wanted to make it up to her by feeding her whatever she wanted. It appeared that there were as many ideas on how to solve her problem as there were people involved. She was bribed, coaxed, petted, and punished to no avail. Val had never had so much attention and she was not willing to give it up.

After a few weeks of struggling, it became apparent that Val was eating no better and was obviously emaciated. The head nurse decided to call a halt to all personal remedies and asked for the intervention of the mental health team.

Although, some staff members disagreed, the mental health consultant decided to remove altogether the gratification Val received and to substitute other pleasures. The plan adopted was to:

1. Serve her minute portions of food without comment; to refrain from praising her for eating as well as to refrain from scolding for not eating; to remove the tray at the usual time.

2. Offer her the usual between meal snacks given to all the children, and nothing more.

3. Assign one person as a consistent mother figure.

4. Arrange for pleasurable activities within and outside of the hospital environment.

Our purpose was to get Val to eat because of hunger, and not for the purpose of pleasing anyone. We also wanted her to stop using mealtime as a way of retaliating and expressing her anger. We needed to show her that her eating habits did not matter to us one way or another.

It was not easy going. Some of the staff thought that the plan was a sadistic one: a form of starvation. A number of people were slipping her goodies just before meals. It took a few days before everyone, including visitors, understood what was required of them.

Gallantly, Val held out for 10 days. It was difficult for her to believe what was happening. She was stunned by the small quantities of food and the seeming lack of interest in her antics. On several occasions she demanded different kinds of food and was ignored; she tipped over her tray and was sent out of the dining room; she announced that she would eat if she were fed, but no one agreed to feed her.

When all of Val's maneuvers were thwarted and every illicit source of food cut off, she surrendered. She ate voraciously. It was difficult to keep the staff from praising her.

Soon after, Val was deriving much pleasure from her outings and from the concentrated attention of one nurse. The eating problem dissolved except when new personnel were assigned to the floor. On these occasions she did attempt to manipulate them by refusing to eat, but it did not work. The staff was finally united on this issue.

FRANCES – AGE SEVEN, ANITA – AGE SEVEN, BARBARA – AGE FIVE

Reacted to Winnie's Death

Fran, Anita, Barbara and Winnie were a closely knit group. They shared the same room for many months and related to one another as

belligerent siblings. The 2 things they had in common were chronic, debil-
itating illness and (with the exception of Anita) virtual abandonment by
their families. Unfortunately for them, discharge from the hospital was not
possible even during short periods of remission.

A major crisis developed for these children and for the pediatric staff
when Winnie's condition unexpectedly deteriorated, necessitating the girl's
transfer to the Intensive Care Unit. Frances was the first to react, by profound depression. She withdrew from adults and the group, covering her
ears at any mention of Winnie. The staff tried to keep the situation open
to discussion by giving the children progress reports, but Frances continued
her silence and immobility. After consultation, it was decided to try
another approach. Because Frances was the most competitive of Winnie's
friends and was seen frequently in argument over possessions, it was
assumed that she was feeling guilty over the events taking place.

Her nurse was directed to talk to her during morning care in terms of
the staff's and other children's response to Winnie's serious condition:
"We're quite worried about Winnie—more than we've ever been. We
don't know if she can get better; we hope so, but it's too soon to tell. Some
of the nurses and doctors remember now that they were so mad at her the
other day. Quite often they scolded and punished her for taking things
that didn't belong to her. You know how she behaves; it makes people
very angry because 8-year-olds should know better. But as one of
the nurses said, 'It's a good thing we can't make children sick by getting
mad and wishing them harm, because it would make us feel terrible if
we thought we had made Winnie sick.' Some children I have known
thought they could make things happen by wishing it; but they learned
better. Wishing is not the same as doing." Fran's response was, "Yeah?"
and a big smile. Variations on the same theme were also carried out by
other personnel. Fran became her old self again.

The next hurdle came soon after Winnie died. The children and parents
were gathered together for discussion. Various fantasies were brought to
light. Barbara thought that Winnie had been punished for being bad; Anita
blamed the devil; Frances said the death had occurred because Winnie
refused to eat; another child believed she had died because her mother
did not love her. A great deal of time was spent in clarifying reality for
these children. We placed emphasis on Winnie's congenital kidney disease.
We explained that it had been a problem no one else on the unit had; that
the doctors had tried hard to help but could not make her well; and that
fortunately we knew how to help all the other children. In addition, we

talked about missing Winnie, stating that she was a friend even though we sometimes were angry with her and that we felt sad about not seeing her any more.

Additional opportunities for clarifying reality developed in the following days. When Winnie's bed was returned to the unit, Anita was the first to speak, "Well the devil got her and you're next Frannie." A great deal of work needed to be done before Anita could understand that the staff did not believe in devils nor were they in league with him. Anita traded one fantasy for another. In the ensuing days she began to eat large amounts of food; this was a complete turnabout in her normal habit. It was discovered that Anita's mother was concerned about her lack of appetite and had told her that Winnie's death was due to starvation.

Fran worked out most of her feelings in puppet play and painting. In puppet play, she looked for missing dolls; and she painted pictures that asked questions about lost people. These occasions provided additional opportunities for reassurance.

Barbara's reaction was to cry a great deal, especially at night. Once she had to be moved into the hallway so that she would not disturb the other children. To Frances it meant that Barbara was also being sent to the Intensive Care Unit. Fortunately the night staff was alerted to the treatment plan, understood the problem and was able to continue the daytime regimen.

It was a difficult period for the nurses and resident pediatricians also. In addition to coping with the reactions of children, they were finding their own feelings unmanageable. Winnie's death created much tension among the staff. There was the undertone of blame and anger that was subtle at first; however, as the days passed, the nurses made openly hostile remarks that indicated they believed that Winnie had been incompetently treated. Defensively, the physicians accused the nurses of overinvolvement and subjectivity. The stress felt by many became the subject of a nursing–medical conference. As a result, the doubts and antagonisms regarding the medical management were dispelled because they were not based on facts. Review of the records indicated that heroic measures had been taken on Winnie's behalf. Once the staff were able to view the distortions in their thinking as reactions to grief and loss, they were able to be friendly toward each other.

The children rallied too. Within a few days, they welcomed another child into their group. Play continued and they were able to talk about Winnie warmly and vividly.

WHITNEY — AGE SEVEN

Had Violent Postoperative Episodes

Whitney accepted admission for a leg graft with equanimity; yet, he expressed some concern about the gas mask that had frightened him in the past. He had been hospitalized previously for multiple surgical procedures for correction of ptosis of the eyelid. All the procedures had proved to be failures.

In preparing Whitney for his operation, both the physical and psychological factors were considered. A great deal of dramatic play was performed with the emphasis on anesthesia. He seemed to understand what was to take place.

On the morning following surgery, an emergency situation concerning Whitney occurred. He accused the nurses and doctors of having lied to him—of pretending to graft his leg, when they really had done something else. He attempted to remove the pressure dressings, splint, and I.V.; he threw his bedpan and urinal at the aides and actually succeeding in moving pieces of equipment to different parts of the room while remaining in bed. He terrorized the children and staff without too much difficulty.

In this immediate upheaval, Whitney was told that his anger was obvious from how he had reacted and what he had done. Since he would not have been destructive without a reason, everyone wanted to find out why he was so angry. Clearly Whitney was confused about what had happened to him because he had bandaged both eyes of the patient doll that was used in preoperative teaching. In addition, the staff reported that his appearance postoperatively was considerably different than was anticipated. A splint and pressure bandage were applied unexpectedly as a measure to prevent damage to the graft site.

He was reminded of what he had been told preoperatively and that his expectations were different; also, that sometimes boys and girls were confused after surgery when things were not familiar to them. He was assured that the staff had not lied to him but rather had not anticipated his appearance correctly and that they were sorry about it. He was then invited to ask anything he wanted to know. He responded by exposing his genitals and waited for a reaction. He was told that he looked all right and that the only place he had been operated on was his leg. With this, Whitney jumped out of bed into a wheelchair, unassisted, and announced that he was going to the playroom.

Later in conference, the staff discussed the clues Whitney had given preoperatively that were forewarnings of difficulties. A plan for future management was:

1. Assign one nurse consistently to care for him.

2. Repeat all preoperative teaching, including the changes; use dramatic play as necessary to communicate with him; make clear the operative site since children around the ages of 3 to 6 are fearful of injury to the genital area.

3. Show him that the staff is not afraid of him; let him know that we are able to stop him if he gets out of control.

4. Request psychiatric evaluation and medication.

On medication, Whitney was cooperative for 2 days. However, there was a second violent episode that was precipitated by a disagreement he had with a visitor; this time, he threw furniture. The staff and patients fled and several mothers barricaded themselves in a room. The atmosphere was chaotic.

This time, the staff approached Whitney by telling him that the law (the mental health consultant) was there to see to it that he did not get hurt and that he did not hurt anyone. Fortunately, it was not necessary to use physical restraint; he immediately stopped his activities and meekly went along to a side office. Once there he related his persecution fantasies to the mental health consultant—how people were trying to hurt him, especially with the operation. The opportunity was used to explore the reasons for his beliefs and to clarify reality for him.

It was important to show this child that people were not afraid of him, and that others were in control. By confronting him with the law, there were external controls now to replace his shaky inner controls. By asking him for evidence to justify his persecution fantasies, those fantasies could be dispelled and the events of hospitalization could be explained to him.

All these measures were palliative, however. Whitney required long-term treatment. Psychotherapy on an outpatient basis and social service counseling for his mother were arranged.

ELLIOTT – AGE EIGHT

Reacted with Anxiety to a Change in Relationships with his Parents

On admission, the medical staff thought that Elliott had pneumonia. However, further investigation led them to believe that his condition was more serious. The findings strongly suggested a malignant growth in the chest.

His parents were informed of this possibility and were presented with a tentative plan for more diagnostic testing and eventual surgery and radiation. They were completely stunned by the knowledge and lost their self-control. In their son's presence they were unable to keep up appearances. The parents were in anticipatory mourning and did not attempt to hide it, nor, did they offer Elliott an explanation for their behavior which was extreme considering the child's understanding of his illness. Instead, they summoned their large family to come from distant places. Relatives congregated and visited with expensive gifts. Elliott panicked and appealed to his nurse to tell everyone he was not sick enough for all that fuss.

The staff attempted to intervene without success. A conference was called to determine how we could be helpful to this family. The following plan was initiated:

1. Assign one nurse to support the parents and to encourage them to express to her their feelings regarding Elliott's hospitalization and diagnosis.

2. Interpret to the family how their behavior was affecting Elliott and how their denials of his perceptions served to confuse and alarm him.

3. Curtail visitors and gifts and reestablish former disciplinary measures.

In a series of conferences held with their nurse, the parents were able to explore how they were reacting to the events taking place. They blamed themselves for the child's condition—for not insisting on a more complete diagnostic work-up when Elliott was previously hospitalized with a diagnosis of pneumonia. They believed that had they been more astute, their child could have been treated earlier. It was pointed out to them that the responsibility for medical diagnosis could not be placed on them, and that most likely the possibility of malignancy would not have been considered at an earlier date by any physician. The medical staff was particularly influential in conveying this information.

By dealing with their feelings outside of Elliott's room, his parents were able to assume a more normal attitude in his presence. They told him that they found it difficult to see him suffer and had probably overreacted to what was happening. The main point was that they were able to communicate with him again. Subsequently they were able to assist in preparing him for more studies and surgery and to give him the support he deserved. Elliott's confusion and anxiety lessened appreciably and he was able to tolerate his experiences with remarkable courage once he realized that his parents would not withdraw, and that his immediate and greater family relationships would be maintained in the usual way.

KATE — AGE EIGHT

Was Rewarded for Positive Behavior

No one could doubt that Kate was acutely ill on admission for the treatment of rheumatoid arthritis and complications due to medications. She was unable to walk and vomited repeatedly. Intravenous therapy was necessary to restore electrolyte balance and adequate hydration. Despite the seriousness of her condition, little compassion was felt among the staff for this miserable child. It was difficult to disregard her appearance and behavior: she shrieked for attention from her mother and nurses, refused to eat and to cooperate with treatments, vomited medications at will and accused the staff of deliberately causing her pain. And unfortunately, the side effects of prolonged medical therapy had distorted her face and body grotesquely.

Although her physical treatment was a challenge to everyone, the emotional component of her illness proved to be the more taxing aspect of her management. A many faceted approach was required. At conference the following plan was outlined:

1. Reward positive behavior (when she communicates in a normal speaking voice, when she is not vomiting and whenever she demonstrates tolerable behavior attitudes) by (a) showing more attention; (b) reading her stories, playing games and records; (c) and giving her the prestige of a special relationship with one person.

2. Reduce the secondary gains derived from sickness by (a) ignoring the eating problem by withholding praise or reprimand; (b) carrying out physical care in minimal time as casually as possible; (c) anticipating her requests and meeting them before she has a chance to demand.

3. Administer tranquilizers to reduce anxiety and to make her more responsive to the positive aspects of the environment.

4. Refer her to the Physical Therapy Department for a daily program of movement and walking.

5. Support and counsel the parents regarding the child's illness and its effect on their family life.

The effects of the tranquilizers were immediately apparent. Screaming stopped and it was possible to gain Kate's attention for short periods. When she was calm and approachable, she received the concentrated attention of one person who provided companionship and pleasant activities so long as she remained sociable. As soon as Kate began vomiting or complaining her special friend left, explaining that she would call someone to attend to her. Then one or 2 staff members appeared to clean her or turn her as quickly as possible and with little concern. This procedure was followed approximately 4 times daily.

Initially it was possible for Kate to enjoy her special attention for about 2 minutes before reverting to the sick role. However, by the end of the first week, the pleasant periods grew to 15 minutes, and it became apparent that the amount of attention she derived from positive behavior exceeded that which she gained from short episodes of self-induced sickness albeit without her conscious awareness.

Kate's parents were eager to cooperate and found some relief in this approach. By this time, they had become exhausted by their daughter's demands, however legitimate. They expressed anger toward Kate for the financial burden and the disruption of family life that her illness imposed. Subsequently, they felt guilty for this anger and tried to atone by indulging her. This action, in turn, led Kate to derive further gratification from the sick role. The vicious cycle was one they could not break until the environmental approach took effect.

Within 3 weeks, Kate's communication improved dramatically. She was able to ask for what she needed in a reasonable manner; she expressed anger toward treatment, hospitalization and having to share her mother with her 2 younger siblings. In addition, she was cooperating with her physical therapist to the point of walking satisfactorily and tolerating her program graciously.

As her improvement became obvious, it was then possible for the staff to socialize with her. She smiled spontaneously, stopped vomiting and demonstrated a sense of humor. Regrettably, her progress brought forth an unexpected reaction from a few of the staff. There was the unfortunate connotation that the approach used in this case denied the child's illness, when no such meaning was intended. It was a difficult notion to dispel and one that influenced future management.

Kate fared well at home for approximately one week. In 10 days time, however, she was readmitted because of vomiting and lethargy. At home, without support, it was difficult for her parents to continue the regimen followed in the hospital due to the stress of other children and household routines. On this second admission, Kate's treatment was considerably different; she was treated in a physical sense only; behavioral aspects were avoided because of opposition to it. Instead, Kate was transferred to a hospital for the chronically ill, essentially unchanged.

MICHAEL — AGE NINE
Was the Terror of the Pediatric Department

Michael, along with his twin sister, was the youngest of 8 children. The staff was mystified by his violence at night towards other patients and nurses. During the day he threatened the doctors that his father would avenge any needles he received for the treatment of a massive cellulitis of the leg. It usually took 4 adults to hold him down for his injections. His language was pungent. He had a deadly spitting aim and was far stronger than his size indicated. Often pilfering other children's night tables, he was once found with a 10 dollar bill belonging to one of the visiting parents.

A small staff conference was held with the liaison psychiatrist at which time it was discovered that there was much known about this family from the social service department and from a city court social worker. It was learned that the father, a construction worker, was violent and abusive; that his mother was equal to him in her pugnacity; and that the older siblings, as each reached approximately 15, got into trouble with the law. On interview, this child told the liaison psychiatrist that he was very jealous of his docile, favored, twin sister and that he often misbehaved in order to get attention. He said that his father and oldest brother praised him for his toughness and would often punch him to show how much tougher he would have to be before he could face the world. Michael said he missed the fights he got into at home.

A treatment plan was made to establish strong external controls on his behavior. The staff was to use force, if necessary, to show the child that they were not frightened of him. They were to resist being provoked into aggressive action by him, but were to be quick in apprehending him with the first sign of misbehavior and in arranging appropriate punishment (with the assistance of his family). It was hoped that after a semblance of self-control was achieved, some tenderness and reciprocity of relationship could be attempted in order to help him learn to be more sociable. A diagnosis of dissocial personality was made; i.e., he made an excellent adaptation and identification with an antisocial family pattern, within which he did have a conscience (albeit it was one different from the prevailing American culture).

An opportunity to implement the treatment plan came soon after conference. Michael attempted to bar the medical staff from his room by threatening to spear, with his I.V. pole, anyone who approached him. His screaming and swearing attracted a large audience. He taunted the onlookers, daring them to come in.

The mental health consultant, who was standing by, asked people to leave the area in order to lessen the gratification Michael was receiving. She remained in the vicinity. By chance, a passing psychiatrist looked in the room and Michael told him not to come closer or else he would be hit. The doctor took him off guard by saying that there were too many trees in the way. This unexpected response so disorganized Michael that he dropped the pole and allowed the mental health consultant to enter his room. When he objected to her presence, she commanded him to get out of the way, stating that she was there to make an empty bed and that he was interfering with her schedule. The boy withdrew to his bed, shouting obscenities and trying to provoke a reaction, but she ignored him. When he was quiet, she told him a story incorporating much of the information she had about his home life. She said:

"You know, you remind me of a boy who was here recently, his name was Giovanni. He went around carrying a shovel. Every time someone told him to do something he didn't like he tried to hit out with it. Of course, he was smaller than you and he wasn't very bright, so we thought he didn't know any better. People kept asking one another what made Giovanni behave that way. Some said that it was because his mother didn't like him, that his father beat him, and that his brothers and sisters were cruel to him. Some people even said that because his family treated him that way he believed that everyone else was going to do the same. That's why he carried the shovel to protect himself. Can you imagine, he thought the whole world was like his mother, father, sisters and brothers! Of course, he was little, and he wasn't very bright; in fact, he was really stupid. He didn't know everyone wasn't like the people at his home."

As she made the bed, she offered him variations of the story. Within a few minutes, he dropped his weapon and announced that he was joining the other children for lunch.

Regrettably, this approach was not well-accepted by some of the medical staff who regarded it as negative and excessively punitive. They sought further consultation from the psychology department for an alternate plan. The psychologist made the alternative recommendation that a kid-gloved approach would lessen Michael's anxiety and thereby enhance his security. It was explained that Michael's behavior was a response to the threat he felt from staff anxiety and anger. Consequently, Michael was taken off all injections; he was allowed to play, eat, swear and wander as he pleased; also, he was given many toys.

The staff divided into 2 factions—one maintaining that the staff's threats and anxieties were being communicated to the child, the other maintaining that the problem lay within the child and his family.

Indeed, with the kid-gloved approach, Michael did not experience frustration. He became angelic and was chosen by the department to be presented during grand rounds as an example of deconditioning behavior therapy. Just as he was to be ushered onto the podium from the backstage room, the large audience heard several loud crashes and a stream of 4-letter words. Michael never appeared. His favorite syringe, which he carried everywhere with him, was missing just prior to the conference, causing Michael to become enraged and completely out of control.

This incident taught the staff that in this case permissiveness had accomplished nothing. The first treatment plan was reinstituted. Thereafter, Michael was subjected to the pressure of a total environment. Once he realized who was in authority on the unit, he became remarkably well behaved and was able to form constructive relationships with a number of people.

Social Service tried to keep in touch with the family to maintain the discipline and direction that had begun in the hospital. After a month of weekly visits, neither parent kept further appointments.

BETTY – AGE NINE

Developed Personality Changes After She Was Hit by a Car

Betty was struck by a car while crossing the street with her 5-year-old sister. Her leg was fractured but otherwise she was unharmed, whereas her sister sustained multiple internal damage and was on the critical list. The mother, an intelligent and volatile woman, let the staff know she was in the process of a divorce, and that there had been many illnesses in the family during the past year. The factor that brought Betty to the attention of the staff was her complete personality change from a sweet, cooperative, almost prissy little girl, to a screaming, ill-mannered brat whenever her family visited. In addition, despite the minor abrasions to her body, she kept the night nurses frantic by requesting assistance while writhing in pain. Because she caused such an uproar, the psychiatrist interviewed her at the bedside, with the staff and her mother standing by. Betty revealed that she fervently wanted to be more damaged than she really was. If she were hurt as much as her sister, this would expiate her sin of carelessness in crossing the street and regain her mother's love. She could not believe that her mother could continue to love her after the accident. She also revealed that for a long time she had suspected that her mother preferred the younger sister, and she believed everyone thought she had arranged the accident. Finally she showed a thinking disorder in which she felt magically empowered to cause all sorts of tragedies and distant events by the sheer power of her mind.

The staff devised the following plan for Betty's management:

1. Show the child the difference between thinking and doing.

2. Question and doubt the fact that Betty had enormous magical powers, and inform her that the way to be powerful was to develop skills.

3. Insist that the things that had happened in the family and to her directly could be talked about with feeling and put in perspective without placing blame.

4. Indicate that others had similar feelings, and that she could get angry at her sister and mother without losing her mother's affection.

By following this regimen, after 3 days, Betty became more helpful, calm, pleasant, less rude to her family, and happy to be rapidly recovering. She did not revert to the saccharine, prissy girl she had been prior to the accident. In a follow-up conference, her mother reported that her emotional change was maintained. The staff felt they had in the short space of a few weeks averted the need for long-term psychotherapy that at first appeared indicated for this child, on the basis of current trauma and long-standing emotional difficulties.

BOBBY — AGE TEN

Resisted Taking Medication

Bobby was admitted for treatment of kidney disease. A rather unattractive, overweight child who had difficulty making friends, he was frequently made a scapegoat. Although bright, he was immature and lacked ambition. One of the chief problems in his hospital management was his inability or unwillingness to swallow pills. Many of the children teased him because of this. Although at first tolerant and patient, the staff became exasperated and ordered Bobby to cooperate, explaining to him that he was old enough, big enough, and was expected to do so.

Bobby responded by vomiting, explaining that he was too sick to take medication. The staff realized that forcing him was dangerous and futile because he was too large to restrain. When it was possible to get medication into him by coercion, he vomited it quickly.

He became the subject of a staff conference and the following plan was agreed upon.

1. Assign to one nurse to promote a special relationship and to support his mature behavior. (He was singled out by Miss K. who played games with him, visited and won his confidence.)

2. Encourage him to express his feelings regarding his hospitalization and treatment; to talk about the attitudes toward illness in his family and

the kinds of responses his sickness elicits from each family member.

3. Ask Bobby for ideas on how his medication problem could be solved. Then encorporate his suggestions, thus making hospitalization more palatable for him.

Bobby quickly responded to the attention given him. He demonstrated the confidence he had in his nurse by revealing difficulties he had in establishing friendships and the loneliness he felt. He discussed the family pattern of sickness—that he was like his mother in the frequency of illness; that his family paid him much attention because of his chronic ailment; and that his brother was not of special concern to the parents because he was healthy like his father. It was clear that this family rewarded sickness, which was also seen as a feminine characteristic.

Bobby's solution to the medication problem was to ask for intramuscular injections. Luckily, it was the alternative measure the medical staff considered taking. This course was agreed upon and Bobby was directed to tell his nurse when he was well enough to change treatment. He was placed in charge. We were careful to avoid a punitive connotation to this plan.

Throughout, his nurse maintained the one-to-one relationship, with the idea of building up Bobby's self-esteem by praising him for jobs reasonably well-done and for mastering new activities. Also, he received a great deal of admiration from the children and staff for tolerating the injections so well. Emphasis was placed on his manly behavior.

All teasing stopped and he began making friends with his roommates. On the fourth day after the intramuscular therapy was initiated, Bobby announced that he was ready to take pills because he was considerably better. He was successful immediately: there was no hesitancy, no vomiting.

Once Bobby found gratification through new relationships and achievement, he no longer needed to gain attention by means of the sick role he played in the family. There was more pleasure in mastery and in his newly found status.

ABBY — AGE TEN

Competed for Attention in a Sick Role

Abby was hospitalized to have a complete and rigorous work-up for the possibility of blood dyscrasias or arthritis. All tests proved negative; yet, Abby persistently complained of pain in her arms. The staff observed that analgesics and placebos were equally effective in alleviating her discomfort, except in her mother's presence. On those occasions no medication helped. A number of staff members suspected malingering. Although Abby was not confronted openly, the staff conveyed their skepticism to her through a lack of concern and inattention. This attitude, unfortunately, only intensified the child's symptoms and increased her mother's anxiety. Abby's pediatrician asked the mental health consultant for an evaluation of the situation.

It was not difficult to converse with Abby once we assured her that we (the staff) appreciated how difficult it must be for her to be hospitalized and to experience such pain. She was told that we would continue to pursue the cause of her problem so that we could help her. This approach removed the need for her to prove her illness. Once convinced that she had a sympathetic listener, she was able to talk freely about school, friendships and hobbies, none of which were especially satisfying for her. At first she hesitated to discuss family relationships, but with help, she was able to discuss her problem. After the birth of her 5-month-old sister, she believed that her mother no longer had time for her and did not love her anymore. The discussion focused on both the positive and negative feelings that family members have for one another and how difficult it is to express some of those feelings overtly.

On the basis of this interview with Abby the following suggestions were offered to the staff and to Abby's pediatrician:

1. Accept her symptoms as real because they indicate that a problem exists. (Once a problem is solved, symptoms may disappear. Attacking symptoms directly may result in their intensification or in a substitution of symptoms.)

2. Focus on the problem. (a) Advise parents to discuss sibling rivalry openly—how hard it is for Abby to share her parents with a young baby; how she must think they no longer have time for her; the negative feelings she must harbor toward her little sister for displacing her as well as her positive feelings; how she cannot hurt anyone through her thoughts but only by her actions. In short, communicate with Abby that she is allowed to say what she is thinking without fear of criticism. (b) Ask the parents to spend time with Abby at home, when she does not have to share them or compete for attention. (c) Encourage Abby to develop peer relationships and new skills (social, scholastic, physical). As Abby acquires more abilities she will rely less on her parents for emotional support and feelings of worth, using instead her own achievements as a basis for self-esteem.

Fortunately, Abby's parents were open to suggestions and were able to adopt the plan. This made additional intervention unnecessary. A few weeks after her discharge from the hospital, Abby's pediatrician reported that she had straightened out.

JILL – AGE TEN

Demonstrated Postsurgical Confusion

Jill was a pensive, well-mannered girl who became a puzzle to the house staff and a trial to the nurses because of her constant crying, screaming, incoherent speech, and angry outbursts for several days postoperatively. The neurologist's findings were unremarkable and a review of her anesthesia showed nothing unusual. Psychological testing showed nonspecific organicity.

A psychiatric consultation was requested. When the liaison psychiatrist saw Jill at her bedside, he noted that she was immobile, had a terrified look in her eyes, and kept her head turned toward the wall. A medical student noticed that from the blinking of her eyes, Jill was following closely the conversation between the nurses and the doctors. On interview, she talked coherently about the happy times of her life: her grandmother's visits, trips to an aunt's, birthdays, parties, and school activities. With any mention of her parents, illness, and events related to hospitalization and surgery, she reverted immediately to gibberish and screaming. Repeatedly, a return to conversations on subjects that Jill did not associate with anxiety resulted in a complete change in mood and greater relatedness.

In the staff conference, it was learned that Jill's illness had brought her parents together for the first time since their divorce, and that her father, whom Jill rarely saw, was keeping a constant vigil at the bedside. The nurses described their futile attempts at gaining her mother's cooperation in preoperative teaching and discussion of illness with the child. They wondered if adequate preparation could have averted the extreme behavior.

A tentative diagnosis of psychotic reaction was made and the following plan was outlined for the staff:

1. Talk to Jill simply and as if she were responding appropriately; to be matter-of-fact with her, chatty and friendly, but when she reverts to gibberish, to tell her that she must be having painful thoughts: that sharing thoughts helps children begin to feel better.

2. Structure the environment by explaining every noise, activity, and staff roles.

3. Administer Stelazine, an anti-psychotic medication.

4. Set up a regular visiting pattern for the parents and explain to them (a) that their constant attendance implies serious illness to the child; (b) the necessity of discussing illness and treatment with Jill.

It was hoped that this approach would direct Jill back to the more usual modes of communication and at the same time gratify her as little as possible in her aberrant behavior.

Within 2 days, her communication changed to the point where she could express anger at her mother. Her mother had withheld information about surgery and implied that only tests would be performed to find out how to get rid of her pain, dizziness, and lethargy. In subsequent conferences with the liaison psychiatrist, Jill's desperate unhappiness and depression emerged and long-term psychiatric treatment was recommended.

SYLVESTER – AGE TWELVE

A Manipulative Hemophiliac

Sylvester arranged for his family to indulge him in every way. This was not difficult, because his parents were in constant marital strife which this youngster exploited to his own advantage. He rarely did homework, never controlled his temper and felt entitled to watch TV continuously. Whenever his machinations failed, he used his ultimate weapon of complaining of joint pain.

This behavior on the part of the parents and child, which was also continued in the hospital setting, so distressed the emergency room staff that several nurses and doctors dreaded being on duty. It was on one of Sylvester's regular 3 A.M. visits to the emergency room, while he was issuing orders to everyone, that his mother divulged the information that the child swallowed any pain-killing pills he could find, even when he was not complaining of joint pain. The home medicine cabinet contained tranquilizers prescribed for the mother, sleeping pills and antispasmodics used by the father, and analgesics for Sylvester.

Curiously, in spite of the obvious maladaptation of this boy and his family, and the knowledge that he was a virtual recluse at home and rapidly becoming an addict, no one in the hospital could muster sympathy for him. Many conferences were held regarding his management, both in the outpatient department and on the pediatric units. For a while, different members of the staff, the teacher, play lady or physical therapist would be able to work with him, but eventually he would alienate them. The staff recognized that he was a patient who was manipulative in such subtle ways that he angered them in spite of their intentions to resist provocation.

The staff discussed Sylvester at a large conference. They believed that over the years he had become a psychopath; i.e., he was without a conscience. Unless everyone in his environment could unite in carrying out a single policy, he would exploit them and obtain sufficient gratification to resist changing. The staff devised a plan for his management. They were to tell him that his behavior was obnoxious, thwart his successful manipulation, use social isolation as punishment for his gross antisocial acts, praise him only for genuine achievements, and challenge his know-it-all attitudes. The social worker explained this approach to the parents. While Sylvester was in the hospital, he became a more pleasant person. However, Sylvester's change in behavior was only a superficial compliance in the face of having been overwhelmed by the floor treatment plan. He continued to be sly, to cheat at games, and to test out new doctors and visitors.

He was discharged in early summer, and for the remainder of the season he was scarcely seen in the emergency ward. The staff were congratulating themselves on their beneficent influence until the usual 3 A.M. visits began in September. It was apparent that no fundamental changes in Sylvester's behavior had taken place.

At this time the parents were seeing a psychiatrist for marital counseling. Cultural disharmony added to their individual incompatibility. The father was from an expressive, emotional family of foreign origin; the mother was from a rigid, puritanical family. Each was afraid to leave the other; yet, they were too bitter to try to make a workable relationship. So far as is known, there has been no change in the family or in Sylvester.

TONY — AGE THIRTEEN

Mastered Fears and Matured During Hospitalization

Following open heart surgery, Tony was uncommunicative and passively uncooperative. In the hope of avoiding procedures and contact with the staff, he frequently feigned sleep or ignorance of what was expected of him. In this he had the support of his parents, who gave him permission in their native language to resist what they viewed as barbaric treatments. They believed that they alone understood him and insisted on carrying out his every need (feeding, bathing, and toileting) although Tony was physically able to manage these activities. The staff felt helpless in the face of the family's infantalizing behavior and Tony's progressive withdrawal.

At a mental health conference, a clear picture of the boy's character emerged. Described as a child who initially made feeble attempts to deal with difficult situations, the pediatric resident added that Tony would give up as soon as he encountered opposition. For example, he had shown interest in preoperative teaching until the realities of the Intensive Care Unit were mentioned; thereafter he literally refused to listen. He was obviously irritated by his family's hovering and at first attempted to push them away or rolled his eyes upward in exasperation; then, he resigned himself to their suffocating attentiveness. Eventually he just grunted or pointed in the direction of what he wanted and it was granted.

A report from the ICU staff (Tony had spent 48 hours in the unit post-operatively) indicated that Tony may have witnessed several emergency situations including the cardiac arrest of a patient nearby; however, he would not mention them.

The staff developed the following plan in order to encourage and support more effective communication and independence:

1. Let Tony know that the staff appreciates the difficulty of his having to accept hospitalization, surgery and constant procedures. Recognize his bravery and talk with him about the ICU; i.e., other patients' reactions in nondirect terms.

2. Encourage him to express anger verbally rather than by negativism and refusal to cooperate with medical procedures; let him know in a bantering manner, that when he pretends sleep, the staff realizes that he's trying to escape interaction; tell him nothing changes when he behaves in this manner, and to bring about change, he has to participate actively in the process.

3. Explain that the staff cannot know what he is thinking unless he expresses himself verbally; that no one can read his mind. Act obtuse when he expects his needs to be met without asking. This ignores his unacceptable passivity and forces him to take a more mature role.

4. Allow him choices in deciding when and where treatments are to be done. Make clear that all treatments have a purpose and that they are not punitive. Ask parents to leave during procedures.

5. Draw him into discussion about his parents' attitude regarding the treatment plan. Offer Tony practical suggestions on how he can deal with his family when they overpower him. For example, the staff person could say, "Tony, your parents mean well but maybe they try too hard, not letting you do for yourself. If you tune out, how will it ever change?" Tony could be encouraged to try saying to them, "That's enough now," or "I want to do it myself," or "If you do it for me, how will I ever learn?"

6. Refer parents for social service counseling as a way of altering their relationship to Tony.

The staff was quite unprepared for the immediate and unexpected response to their approach. When they expressed sympathy with his plight and discussed the Intensive Care Unit (couched in terms of the experiences of others) Tony let forth a stream of 4-letter words. There was little doubt that Tony interpreted events there as diabolical—crazy people doing crazy things. He talked about the constant strange noises, his inability to sleep and his impression of several people beating a man in the next bed and how he kept thinking it would never be over. Once he was able to recount the frightening incidents, the staff was able to put them in perspective, with the connotation of the staff helping instead of hurting patients. The effect of expressing his feelings was seen in his greater tolerance for treatments although he continued his protests verbally.

The nurses' pretended insensitivity to his obvious demands and moods—their refusal to understand his pointing to objects or responses to treatment—had a humorous side. Tony accused them of stupidity—"What's the matter with you? It's water I want, not my shoes." Their only defense was that they were not mind readers. This point was reinforced by his older sister who was a willing accomplice in this ruse. She suddenly developed an obtuseness that was difficult for him to comprehend. When she asked him if he needed help in getting out of bed, he gave his usual grunt. "What's that supposed to mean? I can't read your mind," she asked. In great annoyance he responded, "Why don't you know; you're a teacher, aren't you?" All these occasions provided opportunities to negate the divining power of adults which his parents fostered, and forced him to express openly his feelings and requests.

Tony's parents were bewildered by his newly found expressivity and wondered if it was a late surgical complication. His bluntness was remarkable. It took him some time to refine his statements so that his assertiveness came through without the obscenities which completely shocked this incredulous couple. He needed the assistance of the staff who supported his independence although suggesting more acceptable ways of communicating. Social service counseling of the parents was instrumental in helping them accept a change in relationship after many years of justified overprotectiveness.

The staff wondered what they had unleashed as Tony's sexual preoccupations became apparent. He read "girlie" magazines, pinched and attempted to fondle the nurses, and demanded kisses. Frequent consultation with the mental health team relieved the nurses' perplexity. Discussions revealed that he was merely testing out different forms of expression. The nurses told Tony that although his feelings and curiosity were positive his actions were turning people against him. They told him that he was allowed to ask any questions he liked; that it was obvious that he

244 Emotional Care of Hospitalized Children

was thinking a lot about what was and was not a permissible way to be curious; that although his interest in women was natural, his behavior could easily be interpreted as a rude attack because he did not have permission to touch. The staff pointed out that he had the same right to the privacy of his body.

Within 2 weeks, the beneficial results of the original plan were obvious to everyone. The staff believed that the maintenance and development of Tony's new skills—independence, responsibility and communication—were dependent upon the parents' willingness to follow the same regimen after his discharge. They discussed with the parents the possibility of convalescent hospital care (for the purpose of consolidating his achievement). The parents refused this possibility; however, they agreed to continue with social service in the interest of Tony's continued growth.

HILARY — AGE FOURTEEN

Was Quietly Suicidal

Hilary was 14 when she came to our pediatric department for the first time, but she had been admitted to other hospitals on many occasions because of nephrosis over a 6-year period. She suffered relapses of her kidney disease each time she had a cold; so, she was admitted for intensive evaluation and treatment.

This pretty, redheaded girl seemed unusually apprehensive about the least discomfort and when an intravenous infusion caused her mild phlebitis, she became clinically depressed and began to stroke her hair repeatedly. At first, although her change in mood was noted by the house officer in his daily notes, there was little concern. However, by the third day, her mother reported to the nurse on duty that Hilary was depressed and had mentioned suicide, quietly. Such a strong idea from so mild an adolescent alerted the resident and the head nurse to the possibility that this youngster was asking for help.

At the liaison conference it emerged that Hilary previously had several bouts of depression in the past; each one lasted a few weeks and then left spontaneously. She was the youngest child after her mother had many miscarriages. Her parents adored her as did her much older siblings. The family all lived in the same neighborhood and socialized only with each other. She had never exerted herself in the least to make friends or to excel at school, though she had the modest ambition to be an assistant teacher. This picture of her was put together from information gathered by different members of the staff and offered by the patient while being interviewed at the conference. Her bland, dull answers showed her to be a self-contained girl who felt entitled to having a painless existence and to being unresponsive to the needs of others. Obviously overindulged and egocentric, Hilary was passive emotionally because everything had been done for her. Now being forced to undergo procedures that were uncomfortable and beyond her control, she became furious and saw no reason for continuing to live unless she could live completely on her own terms.

The conference decision was to make an intensive impact on Hilary by undercutting her passivity and egocentricity. This was done on a 24-hour basis by being pleasant to her but talking with her only when she initiated the conversation; having nurses compliment her only when she did something actively; and limiting severely the doctors' generously given assurances. The plan also included urging Hilary to help herself as much as possible and to assist with the younger children, and emphasizing the prerogatives and pleasures of being older and more responsible.

Within a week, Hilary's mood began to change. She was talking of a career in nursing and volunteering her services on the unit. Six weeks after discharge, however, even though the parents were informed of the milieu treatment, Hilary was noted, on a clinic visit, to be returning to her little girl role. Unfortunately, the parents were not able to see prospects beyond her egocentric behavior, her limited ambitions, and her dependence upon them.

ANGELA – AGE FIFTEEN

Was In Search for an Identity

Angela had a marvelous reputation as a patient. We had anticipated some rebelliousness because her condition (subacute bacterial endocarditis) required prolonged intravenous therapy and bed rest. Her recovery was slow and complicated by setbacks. In spite of it all, she remained cooperative and understanding.

In retrospect, it was clear that all was not as ideal as we had supposed. The problem became apparent just prior to her discharge. Instead of displaying joy at the prospect of returning home, she was impassive. Soon after, we learned that Angie was seeking out visitors and staff indiscriminately to recount tales of her complex social life—the numerous substitute mothers she had had since her own mother's death 2 years previously, and her father's infidelities and stories indicating she was unloved.

Two days before discharge, an incident involving 3-year-old Jimmy alerted the staff further. Jimmy's permanent ileostomy appliance was lost.

At first, there was little concern. We searched his personal possessions, bed linens and waste baskets to no avail. We knew there was a duplicate, so it was not a problem until it became obvious that the second appliance could not be located either. Another thorough search was made and Angie who was in the area was asked if she had any idea what Jimmy could have done with it. She wanted to know if it really was important. When assured that it was, she admitted to having taken it and reluctantly retrieved it from the suitcase in her closet. The staff tried not to shame Angie but merely asked her to disclose the contents of the suitcase. She refused stating that it was her "secret sack."

The head nurse directed the night staff to investigate the suitcase as a safety measure. Examination of the suitcase revealed an assorted collection of equipment used in genitourinary treatments—scalpels, needles and catheters—most of which had been denied Angie when she had asked for them previously.

A conference was held and as a result, a number of other incidents were brought to light. Each staff member was unaware that others previously had similar experiences. Angie had demonstrated repeated bursts of anger when admonished for her behavior with Jimmy whom she had adopted as her own patient. For example, Angie was observed feeding him juice with a contaminated irrigating syringe. When she was stopped, she was indignant, stating that the syringe was his own and that his infection was in his kidneys, not his mouth. She added that she could care for the child better than anyone. Other difficulties showed in her involvements with several mothers on the unit and her requests to live with them.

Angela's behavior was discussed with the liaison psychiatrist. His impression was that this young girl had a low frustration tolerance and had not yet worked out feelings regarding the death of her mother. Also that she was in search of her identity. During her 2-month hospitalization she had some stability in her life and had patterned herself in the image of doctors and nurses. Consequently, any criticism of her in these roles incurred her anger. The impending discharge also threatened her security.

The plan outlined for her future management was to (a) praise her efforts in the roles of medical personnel, (b) arrange for long-term psychotherapy through her pediatrician, and (c) to continue contact with one of the nurses after discharge.

Following discharge, there appeared little urgency in carrying out this plan until Jimmy's mother received a letter from Angie threatening suicide. At this time, the liaison psychiatrist contacted Angela's father directly and he consented to treatment without delay.

Further information from Angie's father corroborated the impression that the "secret sack" (a play on her surname) referred to secrets within the family. We learned too, that within her home she was encouraged to have her own way and entitled to do as she wished. She was self-centered, narcissistic and was a party to destructive family gossip about her father and his fiancée. Her father soon arranged for Angie to have intensive psychotherapy. Within a few months, she attained a modest social success at school and was planning a career as a veterinarian.

WALTER – AGE SIXTEEN

Was Surrounded by Chaos

Wally, an overweight, torpid adolescent was admitted to the hospital frequently for the treatment of ulcerative colitis. He was generally disliked because he related to no one, refused to attend school, watched television for hours, and ignored customary daily hygienic routines. In addition, he took pleasure in thwarting the work of the staff with crude practical jokes such as flushing his stools before they could be examined.

Each admission revealed to the staff the chaos which totally surrounded Wally. His parents' marriage was a series of smoldering disagreements. Undeterred by the hospital setting and the presence of strangers, they continued their daily combats without interruption. No domestic issue was too sacred or too picayune to go unaired. The mother, with her outwardly calm and sweet facade, usually initiated the drama. On one occasion she berated the father for having forgotten their wedding anniversary. He retorted that in 20 years of marriage he had only 6 good months, therefore, she was undeserving of a gift.

Wally responded to these episodes with increased bleeding. Staff intervention was required to halt the most violent scenes. The mental health team attempted to decide the best way to approach this family. A plan to protect Wally from the continual parental battles was made with the strong suggestion that mother and father visit separately for short periods. Wally was referred to child psychiatry, and the parents were referred to social service. Unfortunately, they were unwilling to fully participate in casework. Wally's bleeding continued and was no longer responsive to steroid therapy. Consequently an ileostomy was performed.

Open hostility reemerged when the father discovered that his wife had consented to the surgery without his knowledge. The father's chronic peptic ulcer was exacerbated, forcing his admission to a nearby hospital. Paradoxically, the mother appeared calm in the face of all this difficulty.

She compared Wally to her husband and considered them both the products of genetic weakness.

Wally went into a depression after surgery and required daily visits from his psychiatrist. After several weeks, Wally became more talkative and alert. About this time his father, having been discharged from the hospital, happened to visit when his wife was at Wally's bedside. This caused renewed difficulties. Wally became careless in caring for his ileostomy and petulant with his roommates. He displayed a new behavior that was to demand exclusive attention from the nurses and to seek opportunities to detain them.

Because at this time, the psychiatrist could see him only 2 times a week, a plan was made in which the day nurse and the pediatric resident were to use every opportunity to talk about how he felt when his parents fought. From the information he supplied, it was easy to piece together a picture of a boy who had become so preoccupied with the marital strife that early developmental tasks—the resolution of the oedipal struggle with its outcome of appropriate gender identification—never were mastered. All the accomplishments which should have taken place in the subsequent years did not take place; he was like a child of 5. Because he had missed the experiences of learning to get along with peers and developing pleasure in skills and achievements, Wally needed a long post-hospital program in which inpatient, outpatient, pediatric, psychiatric, school and summer camp personnel were involved.

By the time Wally left the hospital, he was helping at the nurses' station, making amateur diagnoses of new patients, and socializing comfortably with his roommates.

The staff's reaction to Wally was mixed. They were pleased that the hospital milieu could be so effective but dismayed to learn that his improvement was not long-lasting because he was not able to hold out against the toxic emotional climate at home.

It became increasingly important to treat the family problem. However, the parents could not be persuaded to seek further help for their unhappiness. Wally suffered a series of complications which necessitated frequent rehospitalization. Eventually, he consented to placement in a convalescent hospital from which he attended school.

BIBLIOGRAPHY

Abram, H. S.: Psychological aspects of the intensive care unit. Hospital Medicine, 5:94, 1969.

Ackerman, N. W.: Treating the Troubled Family. New York, Basic Books, 1966.

Binger, C. M., et al.: Childhood leukemia. Emotional impact on patient and family. New Eng. J. Med., 280:414, 1969.

Browne, W. J., Mally, M. A., and Kane, R. P.: Psychosocial aspects of hemophilia. Amer. J. Orthopsychiat., 30:730, 1960.

Caplan, G. (ed.): Prevention of Mental Disorders in Children. New York, Basic Books, 1961.

Erickson, F.: Nurse specialist for children. Nurs. Outlook, 16:34, 1968.

Fontana, V. J.: The maltreatment syndrome in children. Hospital Medicine, 7:7, 1971.

Gardner, R. A.: The guilt reaction of parents of children with severe physical disease. Amer. J. Psychiat. 126:636, 1969.

Garner, A. M., and Wenar, C.: The Mother-Child Interaction in Psychosomatic Disorders. Urbana, University of Illinois Press, 1959.

Glaser, H. H., et al.: Physical and psychological development of children with early failure to thrive. J. Pediat., 73:690, 1968.

Hannaway, P. J.: Failure to thrive: a study of 100 infants and children. Clin. Pediat., 9:96, 1970.

Korsch, B. M., et al.: Experiences with children and their families during extended hemodialysis and kidney transplantation. Pediat. Clin. N. Amer., 18:625, 1971.

Lewis, M., et al.: An exploration study of accidental ingestion of poison in young children. J. Amer. Acad. Child Psychiat., 5:255, 1966.

Mack, J. E.: Nightmares and Human Conflict. Boston, Little, Brown & Co., 1970.

Meeks, J. E.: Dispelling fears of the hospitalized child. Hospital Medicine, 6:77, 1970.

Richmond, J. B., and Waisman, H. A.: Psychological aspects of management of children with malignant diseases. Amer. J. Dis. Child., 89:42, 1955.

Senn, M. J. E., and Solnit, A. J.: Problems in Child Behavior and Development. Philadelphia, Lea & Febiger, 1968.

Solnit, A. J., and Green, M.: Psychologic considerations in the management of deaths on pediatric hospital services, Part I: The doctor and the child's family. Pediatrics, 24:106, 1959.

Solnit, A. J.: Hospitalization, an aid to physical and psychological health in childhood. Amer. J. Dis. Child., 99:155, 1960.

Szurck, S., Johnson, A., and Falstein, E.: Collaborative psychiatric treatment of parent-child problems. Amer. J. Orthopsychiat., 12:511, 1942.

Work, H. H., and Call, J. D.: A Guide to Preventive Child Psychiatry. New York, McGraw-Hill, 1965.

Index

251

Mental health worker. See also *Psychiatrist.*
role of, in parent participation programs, 62
in staff-child-parent interaction, 91
teaching models for, in working with
children. See *Teaching models.*
Mother. See *Parent; Family, etc.*
Mother-child relationships, observation
of, in rooming-in, 57

Nasogastric tube, description of, to
child, 179
Needle play, 130
Nervous system, central, maturation
of, 20
one year to three and a half
years, 23
Newborn infant. See *Infant.*
Nightmares, following surgery, case
of, 223
Nurse, pediatric. See also *Pediatric
staff.*
and total child care, 3
role of, in psychosocial aspects
of care, 17
Nursing management, fantasies of children and, 12
Nursing mental health consultant. See
Mental health worker.
Nursing staff, pediatric. See *Pediatric
staff.*

Overfamiliarity, of staff with patient,
cautions in, 87

Pacemaker, description of, to child,
179
Pain, postsurgical, description of, to
child, 193
Parent(s). See also *Family(ies).*
alienation from, in middle adolescence, 153
and explanation to siblings of child's
death, 80
changing relationship with, of child,
case of, 229
counseling of, by staff, 77
disturbed relationships with, improvement of, through play, 127
explanation of procedures to, body
outlines used in, 198-203

Parent(s) *(cont.)*
guilt feelings of, in terminal illness
of child, 206
and sibling care, 58
handling of regression by, following
hospitalization, 84
interaction of, with children and
staff, 53-98
complaints arising from, handling of, 64
conflicts in, 61
interview of, with child, 53
of children with congenital anomalies, suggestions to, 85
of exceptional children, counseling
of, 85
preparation of, for diagnostic and
surgical procedures, 135-204.
See also specific procedures.
for hospital discharge of child, 83
response to death, 205-212
rooming-in by, guidelines in, 59
in child care, 57
Parent participation programs, in hospital teaching, 73
and staff interaction, 73
complaints in, against staff, 64
counseling of parents in, 77
lack of parent cooperation in, 75
negative aspects of, 61
role of mental health workers in, 62
Pediatric. See also Child; Childhood;
Children; *Hospitalized children.*
Pediatric nursing, and total child care,
3
and death of child, preparation for,
80
and discharge of patient, counseling
of parents in, 83
approach of, to patient, during
rounds, 87
as member of mental health team,
activities of, 213-249
complaints against, by parents, handling of, 64
counseling of parents by, 77
interaction of, with parent and child,
53-98. See also specific types
of interaction.
role of psychiatrist in, 90
overfamiliarity of, cautions in, 87

Pediatric nursing (*cont.*)
reeducation of, for emotional care, 9-18
resistance to, 14
response to death, 205-212
role of, in psychosocial aspects of care, 17
rounds by, considerations in, 86
teaching models for, in working with children. See *Teaching models.*
view of, by child, observation of, during play, 106
with parents, conflicts in, 61
Pediatric staff-parent interaction, in parent participation programs, 73
Perception, role of play in, 101
Personality changes, following accidental trauma, case of, 235
Phallic phase of development, and surgery, 11
Phallic preoccupation, observation of, during play, 107, 108
Physical examination, of child, cautions in, 88
Physicians, vs. pediatric nursing staff, in environmental care, 17
Piaget, J., childhood development theories of, 20, 23, 26, 28
summary of, 30
Play, advantages of, summary of, 132
aggression in, handling of, 127
art materials in, use of, 117
at child's own pace, 113
books used in, 119
child's view of staff revealed in, 106
destruction during, by child, 121
diagnostic use of, 104
in determining basis of problem, 108
in evaluating preoperative teaching, 109
in observation of child's view of staff, 107
for child who cannot play, 115
for physically handicapped, 116
going beyond child's expressions in, 113
group, toys used in, 126
usefulness of, 109
hostility in, handling of, 127

Play (*cont.*)
importance of, 99
in feeling recognition, 100
in parent-child interaction, 103
in perception, 101
in understanding hospital, 102
interactions of, with children, distortions in, and play, 103
mastery through means of, 121
materials for, supplying of, 112
materials in, 126
art, 117
needle, 130
observation during, chance, by staff, 104
reflecting what child expresses, 111
regression during, observation of, 105
subtleties in, learning from, 105
supplying materials for, 112
techniques of, 111
books in, 119
child's pace in, 113
for child who cannot play, 115
in absence of clues to preoperative concerns, 118
materials for, 112
rules in, 111
therapeutic, involving needles, 130
toys in, imaginative qualities of, 112
volunteers in, 123
with emotionally strong child, 116
Play programs, assistants in, 123
organized, 123
recreation staff in, 122
therapeutic, 122
Poverty, and family assessment, 42
Poverty life styles, vs. emotional health, 44
Pregnancy, explanation of, to siblings, 78
Psychiatrist. See also *Mental health worker.*
attitude of, toward pediatric staff, 92
image of, 93
liaison, and staff development, 91
problems faced by, 94
role of, in staff-child-Parent interactions, 90
Psychological testing, use of information from, 93

This book may be kept

FOURTEEN DAYS

A fine will be charged for each day the book is kept overtime.

GAYLORD 142			PRINTED IN U.S.A.